MW00612111

Unlock the
Power of Your
Chakras

About the Author

Masuda Mohamadi is a renowned yoga teacher, yoga teacher trainer, author, and owner of Radiance Yoga studio (www.Radiance-Yoga.net) in Alexandria, Virginia. With two decades of teaching experience, Masuda has helped students cultivate physical and emotional strength, resilience, and a deeper connection to Spirit. Leading classes, workshops, and retreats around the world that include yoga, meditation, and the chakras, Masuda creates a warm and inviting space for students to expand their awareness, discover their power, and connect with their creative essence. Masuda has a deeply grounded understanding of yoga and the chakras, and she uses these powerful tools to help students experience peace, healing, and transformation. Information about her upcoming workshops and retreats can be found at www.masuda.mohamadi.com.

Masuda graduated from George Mason University with a bachelor's degree in philosophy and a master's degree in creative writing. She has been featured in *National Geographic Magazine* and published in *Washington Post Magazine*. Masuda's publications focused on her experiences as an émigré from Afghanistan in 1980 and her struggles with issues of identity and belonging.

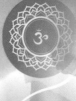

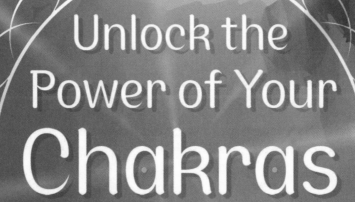

Unlock the Power of Your Chakras

Masuda Mohamadi

Foreword by Anodea Judith,
author of *Anodea Judith's Chakra Yoga*

An Immersive Experience through
Exercises, Yoga Sets & Meditations

Llewellyn Publications · Woodbury, Minnesota

FIRST EDITION
First Printing, 2022

Book design by Donna Burch-Brown, based on design by Winnie Lee
Cover design by Kevin R. Brown
Interior photos by Delia Sullivan Photography
Interior illustrations by the Llewellyn Art Department
Interior illustration on page 16 by Winnie Lee

Llewellyn Publications is a registered trademark of Llewellyn Worldwide Ltd.

Library of Congress Cataloging-in-Publication Data (Pending)
ISBN: 978-0-7387-7102-1

Llewellyn Worldwide Ltd. does not participate in, endorse, or have any authority or responsibility concerning private business transactions between our authors and the public.
    All mail addressed to the author is forwarded, but the publisher cannot, unless specifically instructed by the author, give out an address or phone number.
    Any internet references contained in this work are current at publication time, but the publisher cannot guarantee that a specific location will continue to be maintained. Please refer to the publisher's website for links to authors' websites and other sources.

Llewellyn Publications
A Division of Llewellyn Worldwide Ltd.
2143 Wooddale Drive
Woodbury, MN 55125-2989
www.llewellyn.com

Printed in the United States of America

Acknowledgments

My deep gratitude to Llewellyn Publications and Bill Krause for believing in this book. I want to especially thank Angela Wix for her guidance and support on edits and layout. A huge thank you to Anodea Judith for encouraging me to publish and for sharing her wisdom and resources with such an open heart.

I'm so grateful to my husband, Tom, for the time and care he took in reading my manuscript and for providing thoughtful edits that helped make the content clearer and more accessible. Full of love and gratitude for our life together.

This book might never have happened without the encouragement, patience, and motivation from Jen Mullison and Hillary Lyles Shoaf. I'm forever indebted for the many hours they spent on all aspects of this book and for always believing in me. Deep appreciation for the detailed edits provided by Angelina Fox. To Winnie Lee, whose creative energy, brilliant insights, and detailed edits transformed my writing.

A big thank you to the community at Radiance Yoga, and all the teachers and students who enrich my life daily. So much love to Christy Sisson for taking care of the studio so I could focus on writing.

Heartfelt gratitude for my sisters, Saliha and Maryam, and my dear friends Jessica, Autumn, and Kate for their friendship, love, and encouragement in all aspects of my life. Thanks to my brother, Farid, for building us a beautiful yoga studio and for having a wonderful sense of humor that keeps me laughing. To my lovely mom for keeping me grounded and showing me how to be resilient and patient during life's challenging moments. To my father, who instilled a deep love of learning and service.

Thank you to Delia Sullivan for the beautiful photos and fun photo shoot days. A warm thank you to the amazing Luis Bujia and the talented Marissa Mirra for hair and makeup at Stylists at North.

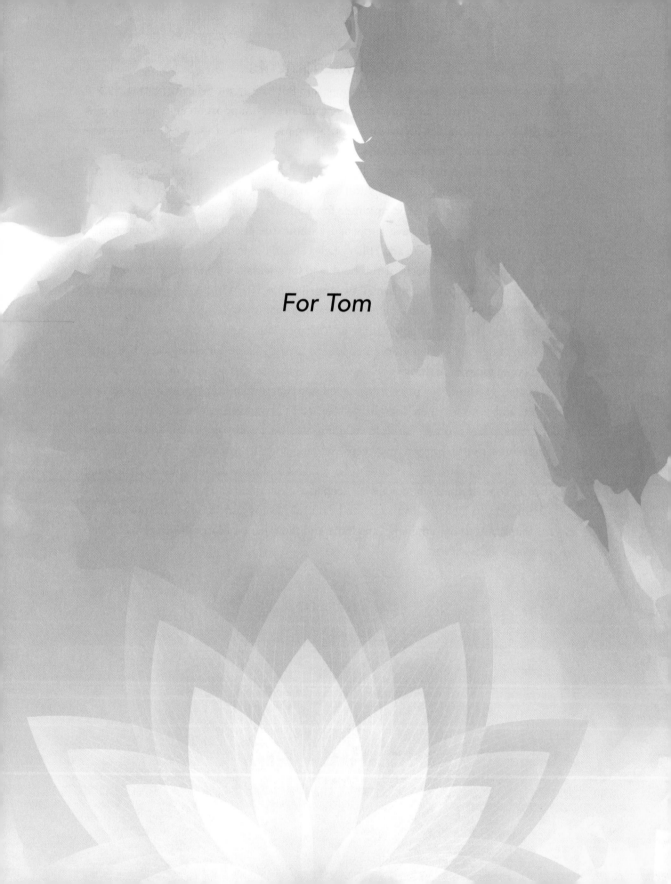

For Tom

Disclaimer

The material in this book is not a replacement for professional medical attention. Please seek the guidance of medical professionals to address any and all ailments. Also, please consult medical professionals when incorporating the material presented in this book into your wellness routines to avoid injury.

Contents

Practices

Self-Assessment

Questions

Chakra Short Practices

Chakra Warm-Ups

Kriyas

Meditations

Foreword

I first met Masuda Mohamadi in one of my chakra workshops at Kripalu Yoga Center in Lenox, Massachusetts. She was a striking woman with a fit body and big brown eyes who spoke with an impressive command of herself. It's been my habit to take notice of people I think have the talent, intelligence, and personal charisma to become good teachers of chakra work, so I was happy to see her again at a later course on manifesting through the chakras, called Creating on Purpose. There, I learned she was not only a yoga teacher, but also a writer. At the time, she was writing a book about growing up in Afghanistan, with a unique perspective from experiencing the war that resulted from America's invasion, and what it was like to be an immigrant in the US. I think it's an important book, and I am encouraging her to use the manifestation principles she learned in my workshop to take that book through to completion.

A couple of years later, she assisted me in teaching the Creating on Purpose course and eventually took all my courses and graduated from my certification program as a Sacred Centers teacher. One of the requirements for graduation was to create a special project demonstrating what she had learned, but applying it in an original way to her own work.

The book you now hold in your hands is the result of that endeavor. Even in the early versions, it far surpassed my expectations with its clear presentation and potent material. I am so pleased that this creation will now find its way to students all over the world to help awaken and heal their bodies, minds, and spirits.

For nearly fifty years, I have taught the chakra system to audiences around the world. I find that no matter what the language, the customs, the race, or the gender, we all have the chakras in common—along with all the issues that go with them. Whether it's a blocked heart, a tight throat, poor grounding, or a fear of taking one's power, the wounds—and the strengths—addressed by the chakra system are universal. Like having two eyes, a nose, and a mouth, we all have these energy centers, but each one's expression of them is unique.

The seven basic chakras provide a map that seems to resonate everywhere, perhaps because it integrates our everyday lives with the sacred and holy all-in-one comprehensive system. The resulting union is the true meaning of yoga, and the chakras can be seen as the "yoke of yoga." They address our bodies, our emotions, our power and will, and, higher up, our relationships, communication, vision, and consciousness itself, all on a coherent continuum from matter to spirit. This map can be used to liberate and free yourself from repetitive and addictive limitations, and it can be used to bring an idea all the way down the chakras, from mental conception to physical completion. Ultimately, the chakra system is a formula for wholeness.

Whether liberating or manifesting, I have seen again and again the way this profound system transforms lives and provides a profound map for the human journey. But the chakra system is not just theoretical. Learning what each of these centers mean and where they are located is just the beginning. At the deepest level, the chakras are an experience of profound awakening on each and every level of human existence, from the mundane demands of living in a body to our emotions and relationships, to the sacred dimensions of the divine.

I believe this experience is available to anyone, but it is only reached through practices.

The chakra system comes from the yoga tradition, and Kundalini Yoga, more than any other yoga style, is focused on practices for raising energy up the spine through a combination of breath, movement, sound, and concentration. Until recently, it was an esoteric discipline taught only by an elite few and misunderstood by many. What has been needed for a long time was to make Kundalini Yoga understandable to more people. This is not to deny the ultimate mystery of consciousness at the heart of Kundalini, but to impart that one need not live alone on a mountaintop under the tutelage of a guru to experience some of the many gifts that Kundalini has to offer.

Masuda bridges the gap from the esoteric to the universal. She has written a book that is accessible to anyone, beginner or advanced, yet she comes from a depth of understanding that honors the roots of Kundalini. The wonderful pictures and practices are clear and inviting, and she effortlessly marries the theoretical to the step-by-step practices that produce a deep and rich experience.

Some argue that the chakras, as they are taught today, have little resemblance to the chakra system conceived of by ancient yoga practitioners. This is only natural, as we live in a vastly different world, have different needs and abilities, and also have a far greater understanding of science and psychology than our ancestor yogis and yoginis. Still, there are aspects of the ancient knowledge that are important to keep, even as the practices and philosophy evolve for modern life.

Within these pages, you'll find the ancient wisdom and philosophy of yoga combined with accessible practices you can do on a daily basis to make profound changes in your body, your consciousness, and your life. You will find information for your mental curiosity, questions for reflection, affirmations to reprogram your thinking, practices from both Hatha and Kundalini Yoga, as well as meditations.

There is something for everyone, and I sincerely hope that everyone takes advantage of this wonderful contribution to the field of chakras, yoga, and awakened consciousness. Consider it an invitation to explore the rich country of your inner world, with the chakras describing the architecture of your soul.

Anodea Judith, PhD
Author of *Wheels of Life*, *Eastern Body-Western Mind*, and *Anodea Judith's Chakra Yoga*

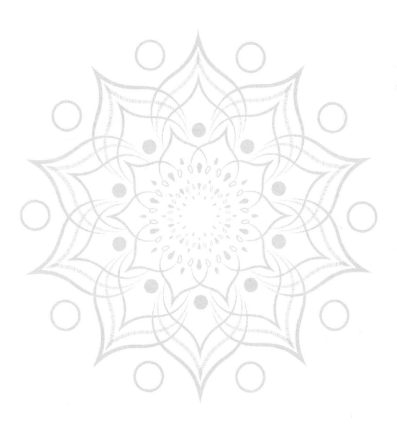

The creative energy of the cosmos
dwells within me and
guides me on this journey.

Introduction

I discovered the practice of Kundalini Yoga and Meditation while leading a writing retreat in the mountains of West Virginia in the summer of 2000. Near the end of our three-week retreat, a visiting teacher led our group in a series of yoga postures, heavy breathing exercises, and chanting. During the practice, I thought the movements and the chants were unusual, but afterward, I felt light, energized, and alive. It left me wanting more, so when I returned home, I found a class and started a weekly practice.

Over the next several years, I became more interested in and curious about Kundalini Yoga, and in 2003, I decided to take a teacher training program to deepen my understanding of the practice. I wasn't sure at the time what to expect, but I was surprised by the experience, because it took me much deeper within myself. As a result of the training, I was able to connect with myself in a real and more meaningful way. The practice expanded my awareness and helped me understand who I was and what I was here, in this life, to do.

During the nine-month program, I was confronted by the many stories I had created about my life and myself, including where I was from and how I was raised. I was born in Afghanistan in 1973 and emigrated with my family to the United States in 1980 after the Soviet invasion of my homeland. Growing up as an Afghan in America, with a strict Muslim family, was difficult, and I struggled with issues of identity. "Who am I?" and "Why is this happening to me?" were recurring questions I grappled with for most of my life.

When I started the teacher training, I went by the name Anna instead of my birth name, Masuda. I had given myself the name Anna at age seventeen when I was applying for a job at a grocery store. I wanted to be a cashier at that particular grocery store because I had a crush on a blue-eyed, blond, American boy who worked there, and I hoped he would fall in love with me. I had noticed him on our weekly trips to the grocery store, and I began to watch him from afar as I lingered in the aisles close to the service desk where he worked. I didn't think I'd have a chance with my Afghan name, Masuda, since throughout school, I had been teased about my name and called Medusa and Menudo.

I felt that this job and the blue-eyed boy had the potential to be a new beginning for me. I stared at the blank line next to "Name" on the application, and I couldn't will myself to write Masuda. Then I had an image of my favorite soap opera heroine, Anna

Devane, from *General Hospital*. She had beautiful, long, dark hair, mysterious eyes, and she was the chief of police. I wanted to be just like her—strong, beautiful, and independent—the opposite of what my family expected me to be.

I decided to write her name, Anna, instead of Masuda. I was hired for the job, and I fit in well with the unusual and mixed crowd of people who worked there. Many were immigrants and refugees like me. American boys who worked there flirted with me and asked me out on dates. This was confusing for me, because I didn't get that kind of attention in middle or high school. I couldn't believe that I was finally fitting in somewhere, and I truly believed that the name Anna was a magic spell that had made me beautiful and desirable. So, I kept the name Anna for the next thirteen years and greatly enjoyed the way this simple change made life in America easier.

Then came the Kundalini Yoga teacher training program, where I was once again confronted with the questions, "Who am I? Am I Afghan or am I American? Am I still trying to fit in and be accepted by Americans? Would I become unattractive to others if I changed my name back to Masuda?" As I struggled to uncover the answers, I thought about my father and my family and how difficult it had been for them to immigrate to a new country and support a family with little means. At seventeen, I had just wanted to be accepted; but at age thirty, I wanted to be authentic and accept all aspects of myself.

The journey of reconnecting with my true self was painful, as I had to work through feelings of grief, anger, and shame toward my family, my schoolmates, and myself. I became aware of all the ways I had camouflaged myself to fit in with others to be liked. The rigorous training days allowed me to feel deep emotions that had been suppressed. I had learned to bury my feelings and become numb, but now I was learning to fully feel those feelings and process a range of emotions.

As I released anger, pain, and shame, I created space within myself for acceptance, love, forgiveness, and peace. Slowly, I released the traumatic experiences of the past so that I could live more fully in the present. At the end of the training, I was filled with gratitude for finding this amazing yoga practice that helped me feel whole again.

I've been teaching since 2005 and continue to be amazed by the transformative power of this style of yoga. In 2015, I met Anodea Judith, who is a master teacher and expert on the chakras, and she elevated my understanding of the chakras to a new level. She has a gift for teaching others about the chakras so that they can be integrated and applied to life in practical ways.

Before meeting Anodea Judith, I found the chakras to be conceptually interesting, but I didn't know how to apply the teachings to my daily life. She taught me how to deepen my relationship with my body, ground my energy, and manifest ideas and thoughts into reality using the chakra system. I had the idea for this book in her training program, and she provided me with the tools to bring it into reality.

This book captures and shares many of the insights and practices that have been most useful in my own life and the lives of the many students I work with at my yoga studio. My hope and deep desire are that these practices bring you closer to yourself—your true nature—and open you up to deeper levels of love and compassion.

How to Use This Book

Each chapter in this book is dedicated to understanding a specific chakra and to you having an immersive experience with it through the exercises, yoga sets, and meditations. The images and colors in each chapter are designed to connect you with the energy of that particular chakra. There is rich content related to each chakra so that you become familiar with the main gifts and issues associated with that chakra. Within the content section, there are exercises that encourage observation and reflection as well as practices to inspire creativity and clarity. These tools will help you create new habits around that particular chakra.

Included in each chapter are questions that invite introspection about your life experiences and opportunities to connect those experiences with the chakra system to discover new insights about yourself and your life. You may discover that the answers you have been seeking to live a healthier and more fulfilling life are within you.

After reading the content section, you will find yoga and meditation practices to bring that chakra into balance. Note that when you work on one chakra, you are working on all of them, because they are interdependent. The short practice section includes a combination of breathing techniques, yoga poses, and/or meditations that quickly work on energizing and balancing that chakra. The exercises can be practiced together or separately. You may practice them several times a day as needed. Turn to this section when you are short on time and need a quick lift or release in energy.

The warm-up exercises are yoga poses from Hatha and Kundalini Yoga to help prepare your body for the kriya by warming up the spine, hips, shoulders, and other areas related to that particular chakra. You don't have to practice the warm-up sets before the kriya. Each chapter has a specific kriya designed to balance the energy in that chakra. The yoga poses, breathing techniques, focus points, and mantras help balance the chakra, whether it has deficient or excess energy. You can always shorten the time for any pose you find challenging or modify it to meet the needs of your body. Make sure to leave enough time for relaxation.

In each section, two meditations are included that work on releasing and clearing blocks related to the chakra. You can practice the meditations for as little as three minutes or for the recommended time. You can also practice the meditations on their own without always practicing a kriya beforehand. It is recommended that you practice a meditation for twenty-one to forty days to receive the full benefits and release old habits that no longer serve you.

Feel free to start at the beginning of this book or jump to a particular chakra that interests and excites you. Starting something new can be more fun in a group or community. If you know like-minded people who are interested in this topic, consider starting the process together. We tend to commit more fully when we practice in community and feel more supported as we start a new adventure. If you are a yoga teacher, this book is a useful resource to include chakra work in your classes and workshops.

Journaling Practices

Finally, whether you work alone or in community, keeping a journal and writing down your experiences as you begin this journey can be very beneficial. Journaling can help you clear your head and make important connections between thoughts, feelings, and behaviors, and can even reduce stress and anxiety.

Guidelines for effective journaling are to write down your thoughts and feelings about each chakra, and also any goals or intentions you have related to that chakra. Before you start journaling, take a moment to center yourself with a few deep breaths and write about what you are feeling in the moment. Use pen and paper to be curious about your thoughts and feelings. Try to write for at least five minutes and work your way to longer sessions. Before ending, take time to read what you have written and reflect on it.

W—What chakra are you writing about?
R—Review and reflect.
I—Investigate your thoughts and feelings.
T—Time yourself.
E—Exit the session with intention.[1]

Self-Assessment Practices

Try the following self-assessment exercises to gain deeper insights into your chakra system and how it's operating.

---

1. Kathleen Adams, "A Short Course in Journal Writing: It's Easy to W.R.I.T.E.," https://journaltherapy .com/lets-journal/a-short-course-in-journal-writing/.

Chakra Body Mapping

For this fifteen-minute exercise, you are going to need blank paper and several different colored markers or crayons. This practice is for connecting with your intuition. Don't worry about your artistic abilities, as no one else needs to see your creation—this is just for you to get to know your chakras. For the moment, forget about the colors and symbols associated with each chakra and allow all colors, symbols, and images to appear intuitively.

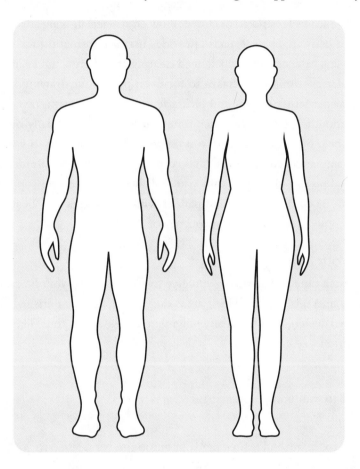

Begin by sitting in a meditative position, breathing deeply. When you've finished reading these next few instructions, close your eyes. Feel the sensations in your feet and legs and connect with the grounding energy of the earth. Then lengthen your spine, bring your ears over your shoulders, and visualize yourself as a channel of energy between the earth and the cosmos. As you stay connected to the energy of the earth and the cosmos, open up to receiving messages from your chakras. These messages can come in the form of words, images, or sensations. You can start at the root chakra and work your way up to the crown chakra, or reverse the direction. Stay present and listen deeply to what comes up. Give yourself as much time as you need to fully receive all the messages.

When you are ready, open your eyes and draw what you heard, saw, or sensed from each chakra. Take your time and let your intuition guide you, rather than your rational mind. Now look at your drawing and notice what you see in each of your chakras. Observe the colors, shapes, and images and see if you can discern any patterns. Which areas feel free and open, and which feel restricted or closed? How do you feel looking at your drawing?

This chakra body mapping exercise provides useful information for you to discern which chakras feel balanced and which need clearing and energizing. From this exercise, you can consider choosing one chakra to focus on from your drawing. Look over the chapter on that particular chakra and pick a few exercises, a kriya, or a meditation to practice for a month. Decide how much time you want to spend daily on the practices and enlist the help of a friend to join you on your chakra journey so you can support each other to stay engaged, have fun, and commit to the process. Remember that the gifts of the chakras are already within you and these practices are supporting you in accessing them. Be compassionate and patient with yourself as you clear and energize your chakras, knowing this is a lifelong journey of discovery.

Assessing Your Life

Notice how much time and attention you give to these areas of your life: physical, emotional, mental, and spiritual. In which areas do you feel most nourished and in which areas do you feel depleted? Without any judgment, assess where you'd like to focus more time and attention.

Physical
Relationship to your body, home, finances, and work.

Emotional
Relationship to feeling and expressing your emotions, connection to your wants and desires, and your ability to deal with change.

Mental
Relationship to taking in information through reading, writing, analyzing, and problem-solving.

Spiritual
Relationship to a higher power or belief and the practices that sustain this connection in your daily life.

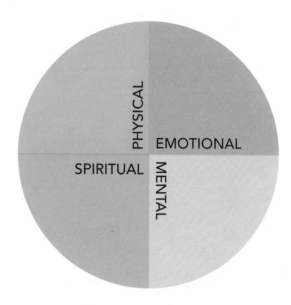

Draw a dot on the line for each quadrant to represent how satisfied you are with that area of your life. Closer to the center means less satisfied; closer to the perimeter means more fulfilled. Connect the dots to create a visual representation of your sense of balance. Evaluate your chart and look for imbalances.

Where do you need to spend more time and energy, and where do you need to conserve time and energy to create more balance in your life?

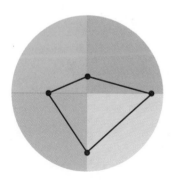

Example

This example shows a person who is feeling balanced on an emotional and mental level, though they must pay more attention to their physical and spiritual needs. The recommendation would be to include more physical activity in daily life, such as walking, running, and yoga. Practice more spiritual activities, such as meditation, prayer, and spending time in nature.

Part 1
Starting Your Practice

At the beginning of any journey, find an opportunity to pause, take a deep breath, connect with your inner self, and set an intention for what you'd like to receive or awaken within yourself. This is one of those moments as you prepare for your journey through the chakras. Take the time to reflect on what brought you here. What is it that you want to unlock within yourself? What moved or inspired you to open this book and start reading? Don't overthink it. Just be receptive to what comes. Eventually, the thoughts and feelings that arise will come together to form an intention for the road ahead.

Once you are clear on your intention, write it down somewhere, and return to it as an inner compass to remind you of your deeper wisdom. As you inhale deeply, welcome the intention into your mind and heart, and enjoy the journey of unlocking the power of your chakras.

Crown Chakra Sahasrara		*Surrender to bliss.*
Third Eye Chakra Ajna		*Awaken your intuition.*
Throat Chakra Vishuddha		*Let your words uplift and elevate.*
Heart Chakra Anahata		*Dwell in unconditional love.*
Navel Chakra Manipura		*Ignite your energy and vitality.*
Sacral Chakra Svadhisthana		*Explore your passion for life.*
Root Chakra Muladhara		*Trust that you are safe and supported.*

Chapter 1
Basics About the Practice

The chakras are a complex, ancient system that has been modified and updated by yogis through the ages to provide powerful tools to bring us into balance and align us with our true nature, both human and divine. In the following pages, you will learn about key concepts in the chakra system. This information will provide a useful framework for understanding the chakra system and how it works. We will explore ways in which the chakras can help you learn practical tools to thrive in the material world while staying connected to the spiritual world.

This chapter also includes key concepts in yoga and meditation to support you in creating a strong foundation for your practice. Take time to review these key concepts to familiarize yourself with the breathing techniques, postures, bandhas (body locks), mudras (hand gestures), and focus points. These practices will help you balance your chakras and awaken kundalini energy.

Chakras

Imagine the chakras as seven beautiful lotus flowers vertically lined up along your spine. Each lotus flower holds a key to unlocking your power and potential. Chakra means wheel or disk and the chakras were first mentioned in the *Vedas*, ancient Hindu texts from around 1,500 BCE.

The chakras are associated with a color, a specific number of petals, a sound, an animal, and one or more deities. The first five chakras are associated with the elements of earth, water, fire, air, and ether. These wheels or disks of spinning energy also correspond to certain nerve bundles and major organs in the body.

The definition and application of the chakras have evolved over the centuries. Current yogis have expanded on the qualities linked to the chakras in order to use the system as a tool for personal transformation in modern life. Ancient yogis lived in caves and forests, spending their days meditating and striving to achieve enlightenment. Our life today is very different, as we strive to stay healthy, meet financial demands, manage stress, and cultivate happy relationships—all while carving out time for self-care, meditation, and figuring out the meaning and purpose of our lives.

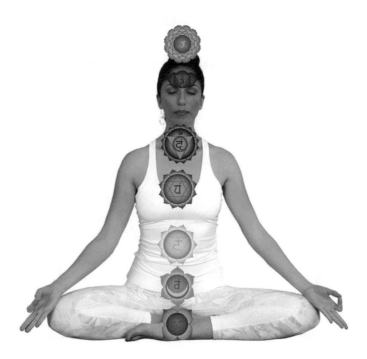

At times, it can be challenging to figure out our priorities and know what to focus on. The chakra system can help shed light on where we are balanced and where we need to regain equilibrium. When a particular chakra gets blocked, we experience physical tension and pain in that area of the body as well as emotional and mental distress. Once you learn about the qualities connected to each chakra, you'll be able to recognize what is off-balance, and apply the many tools and techniques in this book to get back on track.

You will learn to gauge when your chakras are balanced or blocked. If a chakra is blocked, then it can either have deficient energy or excessive energy. When the energy is depleted, that chakra is running low on energy and will not be able to fully manifest its specific qualities. For example, if the sacral chakra is deficient in energy, you may feel fatigued, bored, and disconnected from your desires.

When the energy is excessive in a chakra, it is overactive, and the qualities in that particular chakra are dominating the person's life. For example, if the sacral chakra is excessive in energy, you may filter all your experiences through a sexual lens and overindulge in your desires and passions. Both excessive and deficient energy can have physical, mental, and emotional consequences.

You may wonder what causes these imbalances. The demands of life, and our response to stress, are major factors in how the energy in each chakra gets programmed. Your unique pattern is a result of how you have responded to your life experiences. As you read through this book and practice the exercises, you may ascertain through observation and reflection that some of your chakras are balanced, and others may be deficient or excessive in energy. Now is the time to become aware of this pattern and notice if it's helping or hindering you.

The "fight, flight, or freeze" response is part of our genetic makeup, and it has been passed down to us from our ancestors to help us survive. Our minds and bodies are constantly interpreting life experiences as either safe or dangerous. When we feel safe, we relax, open up, and seek connection. When we feel danger, our nervous system instinctively tends to go into fight, flight, or freeze mode. Think back to your childhood and see if you can remember how you responded to perceived threats in your life. Did you increase your energy and fight? Did you flee? Or did you simply freeze? One of these three approaches became your go-to response to any perceived threat, and that response affected the balance of energy in your chakras.

The flow of energy in the body is affected by how open or closed our chakras are at any given time. Energy moves up and down the chakra system and in and out. The up-and-down current of energy is called liberation and manifestation.[2]

The path of liberation moves the energy upward from the first chakra at the base of the spine all the way to the crown of the head. That is, it moves from the dense element of earth to the subtle realms of light and consciousness. This is called liberation because it frees you from attachment, limitation, and ignorance. This is your ability to see the big picture in life, to align your actions with your values and beliefs, and to surrender to a higher power.

A practical way to understand the path of liberation is to recall a time of growth and transformation in your life. You may have felt stuck in your life, overly focused on the details and your own personal consequences. Once you moved the energy to the heart, throat, third eye, and crown chakra, you were able to move beyond your individual needs and understand that any discomfort or suffering you experienced helped you grow and expand. These are the *aha* moments in life when you finally break harmful habits, stop dating the same type of person who mistreats you, and set boundaries with the friend who is taking advantage of you. The path of liberation requires change, risk-taking, learning new things, letting go of old patterns and ways of thinking, and opening up to

---

2. Arthur Avalon, *The Serpent Power: The Secrets of Tantric & Shaktic Yoga* (New York: Dover Publication, 1974), 25–48.

experiences outside of our comfort zone. Ultimately, the path of liberation connects us with our true self and with the divine.

When the energy moves from the top of the head all the way down to the first chakra, you experience the path of manifestation. This is the ability to take ideas and thoughts and bring them into concrete form and actualize them in the world. A practical way to understand the path of manifestation is to remember a time when you took hold of an idea and manifested it into reality. You received an idea or inspiration from the divine at the crown chakra, visualized the idea at your third eye, talked about it from your fifth chakra, connected with what you love about the idea at your heart chakra, took the necessary actions to make it happen at your third chakra, connected with your excitement and desire to manifest the idea at your second chakra, and then finally actualized it in the material world at your first chakra.

In order for energy to flow freely up and down the chakra system, you need to clear any blocks along the path. The ancients called these blocks granthis,[3] which means knots.

3. Satyananda Swami Saraswati, *Kundalini Tantra* (Munger, Bihar, India: Yoga Publications, 1984), 117–118.

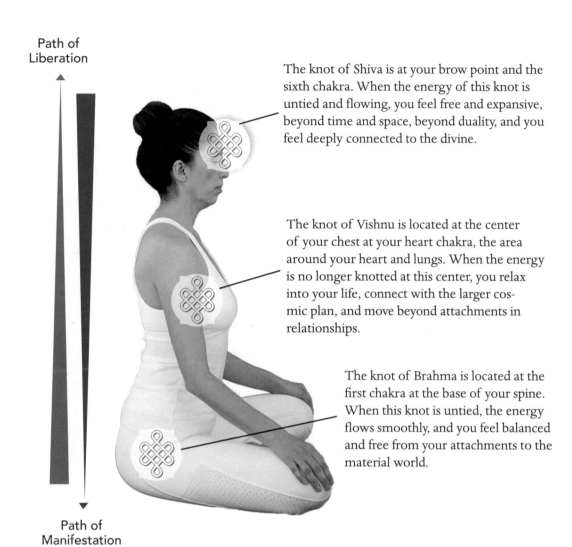

Path of Liberation

The knot of Shiva is at your brow point and the sixth chakra. When the energy of this knot is untied and flowing, you feel free and expansive, beyond time and space, beyond duality, and you feel deeply connected to the divine.

The knot of Vishnu is located at the center of your chest at your heart chakra, the area around your heart and lungs. When the energy is no longer knotted at this center, you relax into your life, connect with the larger cosmic plan, and move beyond attachments in relationships.

The knot of Brahma is located at the first chakra at the base of your spine. When this knot is untied, the energy flows smoothly, and you feel balanced and free from your attachments to the material world.

Path of Manifestation

Energy moves up and down the chakra system, and it moves in and out of the chakras in a cycle of receiving, assimilating, and expressing.[4] These three stages are crucial to keeping the chakras open and balanced.

---

4. Anodea Judith, *Chakra Yoga* (Woodbury, MN: Llewellyn Publications, 2015), 34–35.

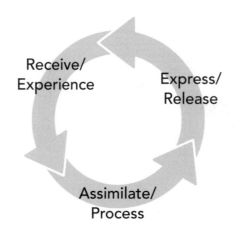

Receive/Experience

Express/Release

Assimilate/Process

Receiving: Your chakras draw energy in through your daily life experiences. Each task and experience in your day either feeds your chakras with energy or depletes them. As you reflect on your daily routines, notice what experiences light up your chakras and what experiences drain them.

> *Notice* if you take in enough new experiences to stimulate the chakras and stay energized or if you tend to isolate and avoid new experiences and then feel depleted or bored.

Assimilating: Your chakra system needs time to process energy. If you are constantly taking in life experiences, the chakras can feel overloaded and overworked. The doer in us doesn't want to slow down, rest, reflect, and go deeper within ourselves to connect with feelings and emotions. There may be a fear of facing what lies within us, waiting to be discovered and understood.

> *Notice* how often you take time to relax and reflect. The chakras need time to process your life experiences in order to stay balanced.

Expressing: Now it's time to release, let go, and empty out with a long, deep exhale. Letting energy out is crucial to feeling light and energized. When we hold too much in, it creates tension, stress, anxiety, and blocks along the chakra system. You can move energy out physically with any activity that moves the body, like running, hiking, yoga, or dancing. You can express the energy out through talking, journaling, drawing, and even crying.

> *Notice* how you take energy in, how you process it, and how you release it back into the world.

Overview of the Eight Major Chakras

1st Chakra (Root Chakra): Survival, Stability, and Prosperity

Sanskrit Name: Muladhara (Root Support)

Symbol: A square with a downward-pointing triangle

Petals: 4

Purpose: Survival, security, and support

Body Parts: Feet, legs, colon, and bones

Organ/Gland: Organs of elimination and adrenal glands

Color: Red

Element: Earth

Mantra: Lam

Emotion: Fear

Physical Issues: Anxiety, back pain, colon cancer, constipation, eating disorders, prostate cancer, and varicose veins

2nd Chakra (Sacral Chakra): Movement, Desire, and Emotions

Sanskrit Name: Svadhisthana (One's Own Place)

Symbol: Crescent moon

Petals: 6

Purpose: Emotional intelligence, desire, passion, fluidity, and relaxation

Body Parts: Hips, sex organs, bladder, kidneys, and joints

Organ/Gland: Sex organs and ovaries

Element: Water

Mantra: Vam

Emotion: Guilt

Physical Issues: Bladder infections, back pain, infertility, kidney disease, menstrual irregularities, menopause, sciatica, and sexual dysfunction

3rd Chakra (Navel Chakra): Ego, Identity, and Power

Sanskrit Name: Manipura (Lustrous Gem)

Symbol: Downward-pointing triangle

Petals: 10

Purpose: Energy, willpower, personal power, and commitment

Body Parts: Solar plexus, digestive organs, and mid-back

Organ/Gland: Pancreas

Color: Yellow

Element: Fire

Mantra: Ram

Emotion: Anger and shame

Physical Issues: Acid reflux, addictions, diabetes, digestive issues, gallbladder disease, hepatitis, liver problems, and ulcers

4th Chakra (Heart Chakra): Love, Compassion, and Balance

Sanskrit Name: Anahata (Unstruck Sound)

Symbol: Six-pointed star

Petals: 12

Purpose: Love, compassion, forgiveness, and balance

Body Parts: Heart, chest, lungs, shoulders, arms, and upper back

Organ/Gland: Heart and thymus gland

Color: Green

Element: Air

Mantra: Yam

Emotion: Grief

Physical Issues: Autoimmune diseases, allergies, asthma, cancer, carpal tunnel, chronic fatigue and pain, fibromyalgia, heart disease, and high blood pressure

5th Chakra (Throat Chakra): Creative Expression and Truth

Sanskrit Name: Visuddha (Purification)

Symbol: Downward-pointing triangle with a circle inside it

Petals: 16

Purpose: Communication, creative expression, and truthfulness

Body Parts: Neck, throat, mouth, and ears

Organ/Gland: Thyroid gland and parathyroid gland

Color: Turquoise

Element: Ether

Mantra: Ham

Emotion: Disconnected from the truth

Physical Issues: Ear infections, hearing problems, mouth ulcers, neck pain, parathyroid disease, sore throat, teeth and gum issues, thyroid dysfunctions, and temporomandibular joint (TMJ) syndrome

6th Chakra (Third Eye Chakra): Intuition, Wisdom, and Soul Purpose

Sanskrit Name: Ajna (Command Center)

Symbol: Downward-facing triangle with a crescent moon above it

Petals: 2

Purpose: Intuition, guidance, life purpose, and connection to soul

Body Parts: Eyes, forehead, and pineal gland

Organ/Gland: Pituitary gland

Color: Indigo

Element: Light

Mantra: Om

Emotion: Confusion

Physical Issues: Alzheimer's disease, blindness, depression, eyestrain, epilepsy, migraine headaches, nightmares, and stroke

7th Chakra (Crown Chakra): Awareness, Expansion, and Spiritual Guidance

Sanskrit Name: Sahasrara (Thousandfold)

Symbol: Thousand-petaled lotus

Petals: 1,000

Purpose: Awareness, analysis, examining beliefs, and transcendence

Body Parts: Top of the head and pineal gland

Organ/Gland: Pineal gland

Color: Purple

Element: Thought

Mantra: Silence

Emotion: Attachment

Physical Issues: Addiction, Alzheimer's disease, cognitive problems, depression, and hypersensitivity

8th Chakra (The Aura): Projection, Protection, and Radiance

Sanskrit Name: Aura (Radiance)

Purpose: Protection, projection, and uplifted presence

Body Parts: Skin

Color: White

Physical Issues: Physical and mental weakness and paranoia

Chakra Name	Location	Organ & Physical Structures	Element	Mantra	Central Issue	Challenge	Gift	Goal
Root Chakra Muladhara	Base of spine	Feet, legs, colon, bones	Earth	Lam	Survival	Fear	Trust	Health & prosperity
Sacral Chakra Svadhisthana	Low back	Hips, sex organs, bladder, kidneys, joints	Water	Vam	Sexuality & emotions	Guilt	Passion	Pleasure & enjoyment
Navel Chakra Manipura	Solar plexus	Digestive organs, mid-back	Fire	Ram	Power	Shame & anger	Vitality	Strength & confidence
Heart Chakra Anahata	Heart	Chest, lungs, shoulders, arms, upper back	Air	Yam	Relationships	Grief	Love	Balance & compassion
Throat Chakra Visuddha	Throat	Neck, mouth, ears	Ether	Ham	Communication	Lies	Truth	Clear communication & creative expression
Third Eye Chakra Ajna	Between the eyebrows	Eyes, forehead, pineal gland	Light	Om	Intuition & imagination	Illusion	Intuition	Vision & focus
Crown Chakra Sahasrara	Top of head	Cerebral cortex & pineal gland	Thought	Silence	Knowledge & spiritual connection	Attachment	Awareness	Peace & surrender
Aura	Electromagnetic field sourrounding the physical body	Skin	None	None	Protection & safety	Depletion	Light	Uplift & elevate

Chakra Triangles

The eight chakras are sometimes referred to in subgroups as the lower triangle, the heart chakra, and the higher triangle. This differentiation helps deepen our understanding of how the chakras work and highlights the different functions of each chakra.

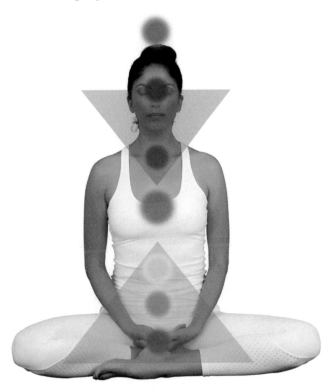

The lower triangle represents the first, second, and third chakras associated with survival, sexuality, and ego. This is the realm of "me": my needs, my wants, my goals, and my ego. The lower triangle is mainly concerned with the material world and is associated with the needs of the ego. It's important to cultivate a healthy ego and a strong sense of self to master the demands of daily life.

The heart chakra energy transcends the self-oriented needs of the ego and cultivates a consciousness of caring about others and embodying the qualities of love toward all. The focus shifts from "me" to "we." This is a challenging shift for many and takes effort and practice. When this shift happens, the energy of the heart connects with the energy of higher chakras, and our thoughts take on a devotional and loving quality. The heart chakra is the point of balance and the gateway between the material world of the earth and the subtle realms of heaven.

The higher triangle relates to the subtle energies of the fifth, sixth, and seventh chakras. The upper chakras connect us to intuition, imagination, soul, thought, consciousness, and the divine. The focus shifts from "we" to "thee," which connects us to a higher power and consciousness. The eighth chakra is the aura, also called the magnetic field, which surrounds the body and is a reflection of our internal physical, emotional, mental, and spiritual health.

Notice your relationship to the different realms of energy and consciousness in your chakra system.

- Are you more comfortable operating from the lower triangle, where you feel more connected to the material plane?
- Do you prefer to be in the heart chakra space and focus on relationships and service to others?
- Or do you love to feel connected to the subtle, etheric realms of the higher triangle, and spend much of your time thinking and imagining?

Ideally, you want to be comfortable moving up and down the chakra system.

Kundalini Energy and the Chakras

Yoga means union—the union between the finite and the infinite, and the union between mind, body, and spirit. Kundalini energy is a catalyst to cultivate this union, to awaken your true potential, and to expand your awareness. In the Tantra tradition of yoga philosophy, life is seen as dualistic, and yoga is one way to transcend this duality to experience wholeness and integration. There is light and dark, feminine and masculine, peace and chaos, Earth and heaven, finite and infinite. We have all these aspects within ourselves and can get stuck in a dualistic mode of thinking and feeling, continually swaying from one side of the pendulum to the other, causing ourselves to suffer.

The ancient yogis outlined a system, or map, to show us how to awaken the kundalini energy in order to transcend duality, cultivate awareness, and experience wholeness. At the heart of this system is the cosmic dance between Shiva and Shakti, a dualistic relationship that has a happy ending.[5] Shakti is the kundalini energy, feminine and divine, and relates to action and matter. Shakti lies dormant at the base of the spine, coiled in three and a half turns, sometimes depicted as a serpent sleeping soundly. She blocks the doorway to the

---

5. Saraswati, *Kundalini Tantra*, 13–30, 81–85.

central energy channel or nadi, called the sushumna, which begins at the base of the spine and ends at the crown of the head. The chakras are lined up along the sushumna, so moving the energy up this superhighway is critical to awakening and balancing the chakras.

Shakti is longing to awaken and to take the journey up the superhighway and unite with Shiva. Shiva lives at the crown chakra and is pure consciousness. When Shakti and Shiva unite, they experience a complete merger and union; the creator and creation become one. Besides the central channel, the sushumna, there are two other nadis that play an important role in our energy system.

The ida and pingala nadis begin at the base of the spine and end at the sixth chakra, the third eye.[6] Normally, energy moves through these two channels without effort. The energy along the ida nadi travels from the base of the spine to the left nostril and is associated with the cooling energy of the moon, receptivity, and emotions. The pingala nadi travels from the base of the spine to the right nostril and is associated with the warm energy of the sun, action, and analysis. When the kundalini energy only flows through these two channels, we remain stuck in a dualistic state of thinking and feeling, fluctuating between warm and cold, emotions and thoughts, masculine and feminine.

To transcend this dualistic state, the sushumna nadi must be opened so the energy flows through all three channels. When the kundalini energy is awakened and flowing through these channels, it awakens and balances the chakras, and we experience more awareness, expansion, creativity, and connection with our life force energy.

Kundalini Yoga and Meditation

Kundalini Yoga, known as the yoga of awareness, helps the practitioner create a deeper relationship with mind, body, and spirit. It uses a variety of breathing techniques, rhythmic repetitive movements, meditation, mantras (sound vibrations), and relaxation to build strength and flexibility in the body, clear emotional and mental blocks, and elevate the spirit. Kundalini Yoga falls under the umbrella of Hatha Yoga, along with Ashtanga, Iyengar, Kripalu, and many other styles of yoga. Hatha Yoga, known as the yoga of activity, is the most well-known form of yoga and was originally developed by ancient yogis to prepare the body for meditation. Hatha Yoga posits that the body and the physical world are manifestations of the divine and are vehicles to help us reach liberation and enlightenment. Prior to Hatha Yoga, the prevailing belief was that only through renunciation and meditation could one reach enlightenment, and that the body and the material world were an illusion to be denied.

---

6. Avalon, *The Serpent Power*, 110–118.

The Three Major Nadis and the Seven Chakras

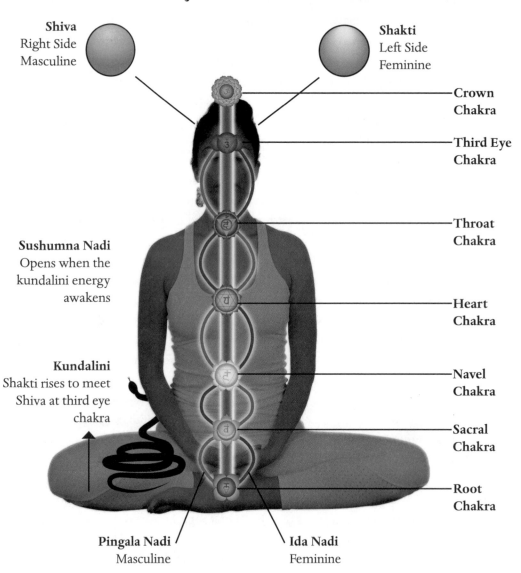

Shiva
Right Side
Masculine

Shakti
Left Side
Feminine

Crown
Chakra

Third Eye
Chakra

Throat
Chakra

Sushumna Nadi
Opens when the
kundalini energy
awakens

Heart
Chakra

Kundalini
Shakti rises to meet
Shiva at third eye
chakra

Navel
Chakra

Sacral
Chakra

Root
Chakra

Pingala Nadi
Masculine

Ida Nadi
Feminine

Kundalini Yoga includes many of the same postures and breathing techniques as Hatha Yoga for building strength and flexibility in the body, but it also incorporates more spiritual aspects of yoga. In a Kundalini Yoga class, you will explore mantras and meditations to connect with the divine.

In fact, Kundalini Yoga classes are unique in that they have a very specific class structure. All classes start by chanting the Adi Mantra: *Ong Namo Guru Dev Namo*. The mantra means, "I bow to the infinite creative consciousness and I bow to the divine teacher within." This mantra creates a vibratory sound that aligns the mind with your higher consciousness and opens you up to having a deeper experience.

Kundalini Yoga classes often begin with a short warm-up set followed by a kriya. Kriyas are yoga poses linked together in a specific order to a create a desired outcome. There are hundreds of kriyas on topics such as improving digestion, opening the heart chakra, strengthening intuition, and releasing stress. Kriyas are followed by relaxation so that the body has time to absorb any shifts in energy and nourish the parasympathetic nervous system, which dictates our ability to relax and unwind.

Relaxation is followed by a meditation to befriend your mind, practice mindfulness, and move into deeper states of consciousness. Kundalini Yoga meditations often include a focus point for the eyes, a specific breath, a mudra (hand posture), and a mantra (sound vibration either chanted out loud or in silence). Meditation opens you to receive guidance from your higher consciousness, cultivates awareness, and promotes inner peace and harmony.

Each class ends with two chants. The first is the Long Time Sun: "May the long time sun shine upon you, all love surrounds you, and the pure light within you, guide your way on."

The second is the following mantra: *Sat Nam*. This mantra means, "I am truth, truth is my essence."

If you decide to take a Kundalini Yoga class, you'll notice that some teachers wear white, often including a white head covering. Wearing white is said to expand the aura, the electromagnetic field that surrounds us; the color white encompasses all the other colors and reminds us of our angelic nature. The head covering helps contain energy in the body, keeps the teacher grounded, and helps focus the mind. As a student, you don't need to wear white or a head covering unless they appeal to you. Generally, wear what feels comfortable.

There are a few other things to consider before you start your yoga practice. Wait at least one to two hours after eating to practice. Otherwise, it might feel uncomfortable to practice on a full stomach. Stay hydrated by drinking (in ounces) half of your body weight of water per day. Practice in a place that is warm, comfortable, and peaceful without too many distractions.

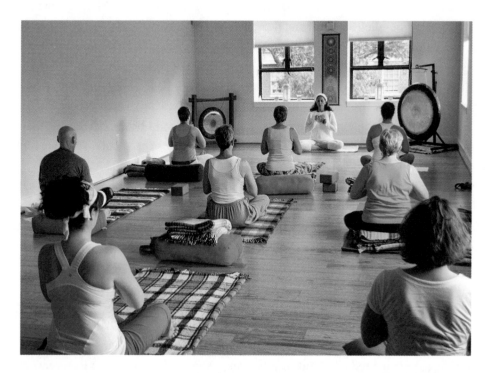

The practice of Kundalini Yoga and the exercises related to the chakra system expand your life force energy, connect you to your true self, and grow your awareness and consciousness. These two practices are powerful tools in living a fuller and more joyous life in which you have a healthier relationship with the physical, mental, emotional, and spiritual aspects of yourself.

All of us have accumulated habits in our life that serve us and habits that don't. The chakra system brings awareness to these habits, and the practice of Kundalini Yoga energizes and elevates you, so you commit to the habits that serve you and break free from the habits that derail you.

Yoga Basics

Awareness about your breath, posture, and alignment can have enormous benefits in your daily life. Your breath is directly linked to your energy, vitality, and mental clarity. Your posture, the way you sit and stand, affects how energy moves and flows through your body. Sometimes it's the obvious, simple changes that can have the most profound impacts.

Your Relationship to Your Breath

The length and depth of your breath is linked to your energy and mood. Yogic breathing techniques help return the body to a more relaxed state, release armoring from prolonged tension, and increase the flow of prana (life-giving energy). The movement of prana through the nadis determines our level of energy and vitality.

Long, Deep Breathing

Practice long, deep breathing either lying on your back or sitting on the floor or in a chair. If lying down, make sure you are comfortable and, if needed, bend your knees and keep your feet flat on the floor. If sitting up, make sure the spine is long and straight with your head over your heart and your heart over the belly button.

Inhale through your nose and expand your abdomen, then your chest and the area around the collarbone. Exhale through your nose and relax the collarbone and chest and then pull the abdomen in toward the spine. Notice the sensations in the back of the body as you breathe. Visualize your abdominal and chest area expanding like a balloon in all directions on the inhale and releasing on the exhale.

Continue at your own pace and slow down the inhalation and exhalation as much as you can. Keep breathing in through the nose to filter the air before it moves into the lungs. Aim for a three- to five-second inhale and a three- to five-second exhale.

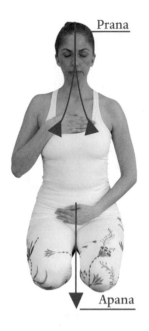

Prana

Apana

Prana and Apana

In yogic terms, the inhale brings in prana, giving you energy and vitality. Prana expands your capacity for life. The exhale releases apana, which is the energy of elimination. Apana allows you release what you no longer need.

Benefits of long, deep breathing: increases oxygen intake, reduces and prevents the buildup of toxins in the lungs, cleanses the blood, and calms and relaxes the nervous system.

Breath of Fire

Once you're comfortable with long, deep breathing, begin practicing breath of fire. Many Kundalini Yoga sets use this powerful breath. It's a rapid, rhythmic, and continuous breath powered from the navel point.

The navel point is the area a few inches below the belly button and believed to be the seat of vital energy and power. The yogis believe that seventy-two thousand nadis meet at the navel point.

The inhale and exhale are equal in length and strength, and about two to three cycles per second (as if a dog were panting rapidly). Beginners may start with a slower cycle. On the inhale, gently relax the navel area and diaphragm. While exhaling, gently pull the navel and diaphragm up. If you find that you are running out of breath, slow down the rhythm. Make sure the inhale and exhale are equal in length. This is not kalabbati breathing, which emphasizes a more powerful exhale.

Benefits of breath of fire: releases toxins from the lungs, mucous lining, blood vessels, and cells; expands lung capacity and strengthens the navel point.

Posture

Once you've understood the breath, it's time to notice how you sit and stand. The yogis believe that your posture affects the flow of energy in your body. Maintaining the natural curve of your spine while sitting and standing improves your posture and allows the energy to flow through all the chakras. Ideally your head is balanced over your heart and your heart is over your navel point. It is recommended that you stay connected to and move from the navel point during your yoga practice and during your daily activities.

Notice if you prefer to walk and sit with your head leaning forward. Or do you curve your spine forward, causing undue strain on your low back? Start by paying attention to how you sit and stand and how this feels in your body. Then start to make minor adjustments to bring your body back into balance.

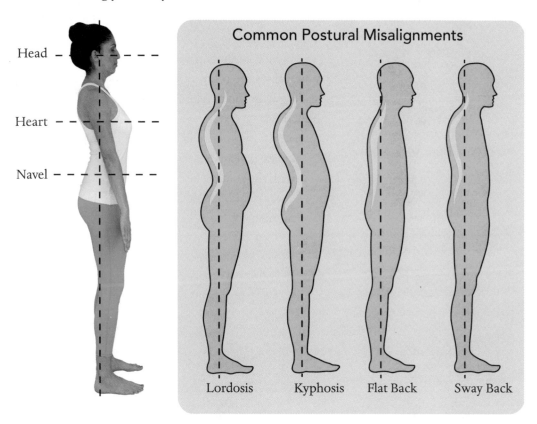

Head – – – – – –

Heart – – – – – –

Navel – – – – – –

Common Postural Misalignments

Lordosis Kyphosis Flat Back Sway Back

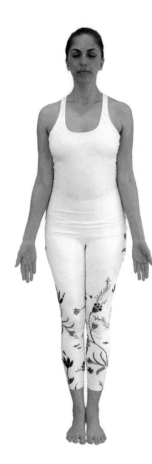

Mountain Pose

Stand with the feet together or hip-distance apart. Distribute the weight evenly on both feet. Soften the knees. Gently pull the abdomen in and lift the chest. Relax the shoulders away from the ears. Let the arms hang down with the palms facing forward. Visualize a golden ray of light moving from the base of the spine down into the depths of the earth to ground your energy. Visualize another golden ray of light moving from the top of your head up toward the sky, connecting you to spirit. Visualize yourself as a channel for the energy of the earth and the ethers.

Practice mountain pose for one minute, then walk across the room in a slow, deliberate manner, leading with the navel point. Notice how it feels to walk this way.

Benefits: Improves posture; strengthens thighs, knees, and ankles; deepens connection with the root chakra; invites grounding energy; and cultivates awareness to be in the moment.

Easy Pose

Sit with a straight spine, connect with your navel point, and relax your shoulders. Either cross the ankles or place one foot in front of the other. The knees are relaxed and below the hips. If the knees are higher than the hips, sit on a blanket for additional support.

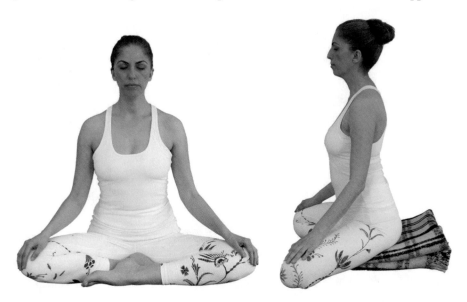

Benefits: Stimulates the pelvis, spine, and abdomen; stretches the ankles and knees; and keeps the mind alert.

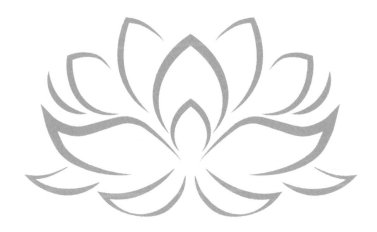

Rock Pose

Sit on your heels with a straight spine. The heels are pressing into the center of each buttock. If this is painful on your knees or ankles, sit on a block or blanket. If it's still painful, better to practice easy pose instead.

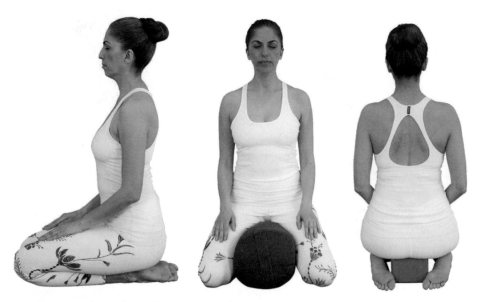

Benefits: Stimulates digestion.

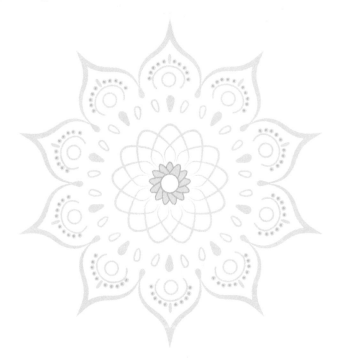

Bandhas

Bandhas, or body locks, direct prana and apana, the generative and eliminating energies. The bandhas are a combination of muscle contractions that direct the flow of energy and change blood circulation. Bandhas also help break or untie the three major granthis or knots along the chakras system.

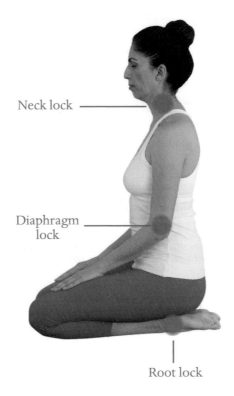

Neck lock

Diaphragm lock

Root lock

The Great Lock/Mahabandha

Mahabandha is the application of all three locks at the same time with your breath held out.

> *Benefits:* When the great lock is applied consciously and correctly, the body is said to enter a healing state of balance. Yogic tradition tells us that the healing effects of this lock may help with menstrual cramps, poor circulation, and preoccupation with mental fantasies.

Neck Lock/Jalandhar Bandha

Neck lock is the most basic and generally applied lock. It regulates the movement of energy in the upper part of the body. Neck lock is practiced during all meditations.

In neck lock, lift the chest and sternum up while lengthening the back of the neck and pulling the chin in slightly. The neck, throat, and face muscles remain relaxed. Keep the ears over the shoulders.

> *Benefits:* Regulates blood pressure, minimizes external distractions, seals energy in the brain stem, and directs pranic energy into the central channel to calm the heart.

Diaphragm Lock/Uddiyana Bandha

Make sure to practice on an empty stomach. Apply this lock only with your breath fully exhaled, holding your breath out. Inhale deeply and exhale completely through the nose. Hold the breath out. Pull your entire abdominal region, especially the area above your belly button, back toward your spine. Keep your chest lifted and do not allow your chest to collapse downward. Press the lower thoracic spine forward gently.

Keep the lift strongly applied for ten to sixty seconds, according to your ability, without strain, and maintain a concentrated sense of calm. Release the lock by relaxing your abdomen and gradually inhaling.

> *Benefits:* Helps strengthen your digestion by increasing the fire element, the element of transformation, in your abdominal region. Opens the flow of energy to your heart chakra and enhances your ability to be sensitive, compassionate, and kind.

Root Lock/Mula Bandha

Root lock coordinates, stimulates, and balances the energies involved with the rectum, sex organs, and navel point.

In one smooth, rapid motion, contract the muscles around the perineum, the sex organ, the muscles of the lower abdomen, and pull in and up on the navel point. Root lock can be applied on the inhale or exhale.

> *Benefits:* Blends prana and apana at the navel point, which opens the entrance to the sushumna for energy to flow up the spine. Stimulates the proper flow of spinal fluid and crystalizes the effects of a pose.

Mudras

Kundalini Yoga uses different hand postures to activate pressure points that help energy flow along the meridians of the brain. This activation clears the subconscious mind and allows access to the higher centers of the brain.

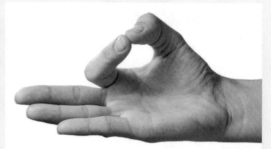

Gyan Mudra (Seal of Wisdom)
Touch the tip of the index finger and the tip of the thumb together. The other three fingers are straight. Gyan mudra stimulates knowledge, wisdom, receptivity, expansion, and calmness.

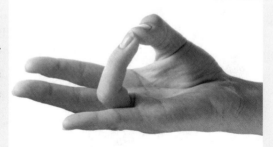

Shuni Mudra (Seal of Patience)
Touch the tip of the middle finger and the tip of the thumb together. The other three fingers are straight. Shuni mudra promotes patience, discernment, courage, and commitment.

Surya Mudra (Seal of Sun)
Touch the tip of the ring finger and the tip of the thumb together. The other three fingers are straight. Surya mudra revitalizes energy, nerve strength, health, and sexuality.

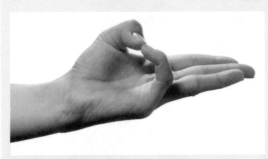

Buddhi Mudra (Seal of Mental Clarity)

Touch the tip of the little finger and the tip of the thumb together. The other three fingers are straight. Buddhi mudra creates the capacity to clearly and intuitively communicate as well as stimulates psychic development and mental powers of communication.

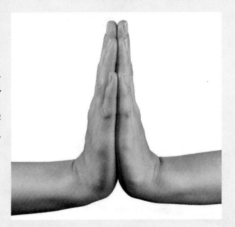

Prayer Pose

The palms of both hands and fingers are completely touching. The outer edge of the mound of the thumb is pressed into the sternum. Prayer pose neutralizes the right and left side of the body connected with the masculine and feminine energies.

Venus Mudra

To connect with your masculine energy, interlace the fingers with the left little finger on the bottom. Place the left thumb in the webbing between the thumb and index finger of the right hand. The right thumb presses the fleshy mound at the base of the left thumb.

To connect with your feminine energy, the thumb positions are reversed, and the right little finger goes on the bottom. Venus mudra channels sexual energy, promotes glandular balance, and improves your ability to concentrate more easily.

Focus Points

Kundalini Yoga and Meditation use different focus points to deepen your awareness, to be in the present moment, and to connect with the higher centers of consciousness. Different focus points are used in different meditations in this book.

Crown Center

The eyes are closed and rolled upward toward the crown. The crown center stimulates the pineal gland and invites feelings of elevation and expansion.

Third Eye Point

Focus at the top of the nose between the eyebrows. The eyes are closed and look upward and inward. The third eye point stimulates the pituitary gland and develops intuition.

Lotus Point

The eyes are slightly open and looking down at the tip of the nose. The lotus point controls the mind, stimulates the frontal lobe, and develops intuition.

Moon Center

The eyes are closed and focus downward toward the chin. Focusing at the moon center is cooling and calming for the emotions and provides insights to see yourself more clearly.

Mantras

Mantras are chants that create subtle vibrations that can elevate consciousness. Chanting mantras helps focus the mind during meditation, especially for new students. It can be overwhelming to sit quietly in meditation and simply observe your thoughts, so concentrating on a mantra can make the transition to silent meditation easier.

Mantras alter the patterns of the mind by stimulating the eighty-four meridian points, or pressure points, in the roof of the mouth. Every time you speak, your tongue taps and stimulates them, along with their associated glands and organs. Every time you chant a mantra, you tap a particular sequence and rhythm that initiates these reactions in the brain and body.

Mantras also work on cutting through the limitations of the ego to expand the mind and to connect you with the sacred within. While the origins of mantras are from the religious traditions of India, you don't need to practice any religion to receive the benefits of the mantras, as the sound vibrations have a universal healing effect on everyone.

Many of the meditations in this book use mantras to help alleviate anxiety and fear, cultivate peace of mind, and increase intuition. Over time, you may come to rely on the mantras in your daily life to create more ease and calm. At first, you may feel self-conscious about your voice, but know that chanting is not singing. Chanting is opening yourself up to the universe and aligning your vibration with the vibration of the cosmos. Over time, you may fall in love with the sound of your voice as you connect with the beauty of it.

Part 2
The Lower Triangle

The lower triangle, which includes chakras one, two, and three, is the realm of self-orientation and self-motivation. The three chakras in the lower triangle have to do with our life on Earth and relate to our survival, our feelings and desires, and our ego and power.

The first chakra is our foundation; it relates to our survival, security, body, health, and prosperity. When chakra one is balanced, we are at ease with our day-to-day life and have created a safe and comfortable existence where our needs are met. We feel safe in the world, trust the process of life, and feel healthy. After the needs of the first chakra are met, we can sit back and enjoy life and connect with the things that bring us pleasure.

The second chakra is our relationship to desire, feelings, joy, fun, and relaxation. Chakra two also gives us access to our emotions and our ability to slow down enough in life to feel our feelings. When chakra two is balanced, we are tuned in to our feelings, able to relax and enjoy life. Feeling nourished and nurtured, we know that we are enough just as we are.

The third chakra is the seat of our energy, vitality, and power. This is the chakra that gets things done, accomplishes, and builds a strong sense of self. It's the doer in us. When chakra three is balanced, we are energized, strong, and courageous, and we follow through on our commitments.

The lower chakras connect us with our human nature, our habits and impulses, and the needs of our ego related to self-promotion and self-protection. A strong, balanced lower triangle creates the foundation for the entire chakra system.

Trust that you are safe and supported.

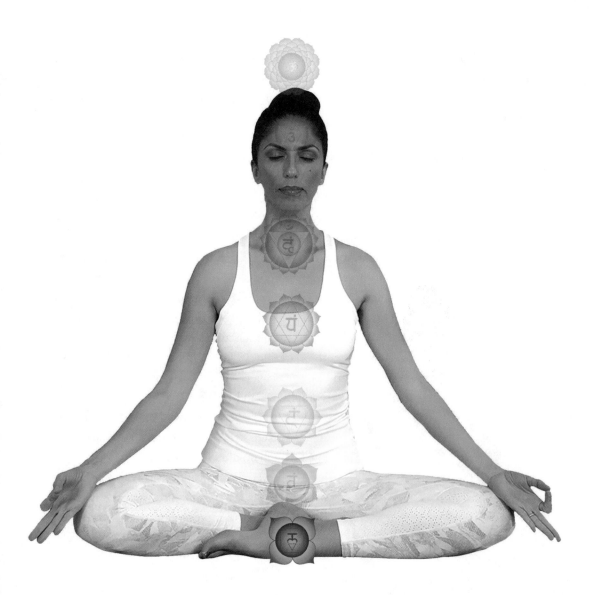

Chapter 2
ROOT CHAKRA (1st Chakra)

Sanskrit Name: Muladhara (Root Support)

Main Issues: Survival, health, prosperity, and fear

Element: Earth

Location: At the perineum, between the genitals and anus at the base of the spine

Color: Red

Goals: A strong and healthy body, good management of finances, fulfilling work, sense of safety, and trust in the world

Balanced Energy

- Grounded
- Physically healthy
- Connected to body
- Stable and secure
- Prosperous attitude
- Ability to be present
- Ability to manifest and finish tasks

Deficient Energy

- Fearful
- Anxious
- Spacey
- Restless
- Undereating
- Disconnected from body
- Difficulty completing tasks

Excessive Energy

- Sluggish
- Resistant to change
- Material fixation
- Hoarding
- Overeating
- Greedy
- Stubborn

Healing Practices

Spend time in nature hiking or gardening

Pay attention to the food you're consuming

Move the body with exercise and yoga

Slow down and pay attention to the details of your life

Track your spending

Get a massage

Affirmations

I love life and am grateful to be here.

I'm grounded in my body and I live in the moment.

My body supports me in living a creative and happy life.

It is safe for me to be here.

I'm connected to Mother Earth and am open to receiving.

I'm open to prosperity in all aspects of my life.

The Symbol

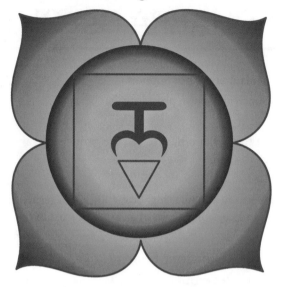

The chakra one symbol is depicted as a circle with four outer petals. The four petals represent the four forms of bliss: joy, natural pleasure, delight in controlling passion, and blissfulness in concentration. The four petals can also be said to symbolize four aspects of consciousness: mind, intellect, consciousness, and ego.

Inside the circle is a yellow square, which represents the number four and relates to the four elements and the four seasons. The inverted triangle within the square represents the kundalini energy and the tripurna, the three worlds, which represent the three divinities: Brahma, Vishnu, and Shiva.

Some versions of the symbol will include an elephant inside the square with seven trunks to signify strength and patience. The seed sound is **Lam.**

Relationship to Earth

One way to bring more healing to the root chakra is to write a beautiful welcome message from yourself to your inner child:

Welcome to the world.
I'm so glad you are here.
You are beautiful, unique, and deeply loved.

The earth is our foundation and offers us the stable and solid ground we need to feel rooted and grounded while continually growing and evolving. Take a moment to notice how safe and secure you feel in the world. Do you feel you belong here and deserve to be here? Do you trust the world to keep you safe and support you in your life?

Yogis believe that the first forty days of life impact the energy at our root chakra because we are separated from the safety of the mother's womb and enter a new realm of change and uncertainty. If, during those first forty days, we are kept in constant contact with our mother, loved and nurtured, then a sense of connection and emotional security develops in the root chakra. If we didn't have this experience as infants, we may need to nourish the energy at our root chakra by practicing yoga, meditation, and some healing visualizations.

One of our main challenges is to transcend the experience of separation and uncertainty at birth and learn to trust the earth, ourselves, and life. When we don't trust, the energy flow at the root chakra either constricts or stops flowing, and we can lose touch with ourselves and the healing energy of the earth.

Relationship to Your Home

Take a moment and visualize your home.

How does it reflect who you are?
Does it feel safe and comfortable?
Does it nurture you?
Do you spend too little time,
     enough time, or too much time at home?

Your home is a place to feel safe and comfortable, a sanctuary to disconnect from the demands of the world, and a place to relax and create loving memories with family, friends, and pets.

Your home reflects your root chakra. The root chakra wants you to feel safe, stable, and secure, and your home is a place to experience this sense of safety. Making your home a clean, comfortable, and nurturing place replenishes the root chakra with healing energy. Take time to declutter your home and finish projects, because incomplete projects and disorder drain your energy and can weaken the root chakra. Enlist the help of others if this seems like a daunting task. Either hire a professional or barter with your friends to help you clean out your closet, your garage, and the kitchen drawers.

Closets are a great place to get started with clearing clutter. Try on all your clothes and organize them into three piles: keep it, give it away, and throw it away. If this feels overwhelming, enlist the help of friends who will help you make decisions because they're not attached to your prom dress from high school. Once you've organized your piles, make sure to drop off the bags at your local thrift store or charity. Otherwise, those bags may sit in the closet, garage, or the back of your car for weeks or even months. The drop-off completes the cycle, and then you can sit back and enjoy your clutter-free space.

Relationship to Your Body

Take a moment and pay close attention to your body.

What do you notice?
How do you feel about your body?
How do you feel in your body?
What would it take to accept and appreciate your body as it is in this moment?

The body is your vehicle; it allows you to experience life and is the foundation for the chakra system. Exercise, healthy eating, sleeping enough, and going to the doctor as needed are critical to maintaining a balanced root chakra and relationship with your body. If this relationship is neglected, imbalances can occur that lead to chronic health issues, poor posture, low energy, and resistance to taking care of basic needs in your life.

Slowing down, paying attention to your body, and adopting a loving attitude toward yourself can have many healing benefits for your root chakra.

Your body is a teacher that lets you know when you are out of balance. Throughout the day, check in with your body, listen to the subtle sensations and messages, and make the necessary changes to create more ease and balance. Include a twenty-minute walk into your daily routine and make sure to take five-minute stretch breaks at your desk throughout the day.

Relationship to Money

Bring your awareness to your relationship with money.

Do you have enough for the basics?
Do you attract money but then spend it all?
Do you have plenty but don't feel satisfied?

Our relationship with money can be complex and complicated as it relates to our ability to survive and thrive in life. Internal and external conflicts about money can evoke strong emotions and tap into our values and beliefs.

Money is related to the root chakra because you need money to survive, pay your bills, live in your home, and travel from place to place. People who have difficulty with money often have difficulty being organized and paying attention to the details. The root chakra requires that you pay attention to how much you spend and what you spend it on, and that you create a budget.

For one month, monitor your spending and write down every expense. What do you spend your money on? Does your income cover your expenses? If not, how can you either increase your income or decrease your spending? Changing your relationship with money requires paying attention to the details and facing the facts. Notice what you notice about your spending and saving habits and see if you can create healthier patterns that support you in your financial goals.

Notice if any of these beliefs resonate with you:

Money corrupts. Money is evil.   I'll never have money.
I'm not good at managing money.   I can't save money.
   Did you learn any of these beliefs from your family?

Practice replacing negative beliefs with more positive ones and practice the new beliefs daily:

Money is freedom.   Money is a useful resource that I invite into my life.
I deserve to be wealthy.   Wealth flows to me from every direction.

Relationship to Manifestation and Prosperity

> Consider how you manifest the things you want in life.
>
> *Are you someone who completes and finishes projects?*
>
> *Do you feel safe in the world and trust the process of life?*
>
> *Are you connected to your life purpose and what truly makes you happy?*

Chakras are powerful tools in helping us manifest ideas into realities and feeling prosperous regardless of external circumstances. The root chakra is key to manifesting any idea or dream in your life. The root chakra is where you complete the final steps to any dream or project and bring the final product into being. Completing these final steps takes patience, commitment, and attention to details. Manifestation is about finding and organizing the resources you need to fulfill a dream.

In pursuing a dream, you can have an attitude of scarcity, abundance, or prosperity. Scarcity is the attitude that there isn't enough in the world for everyone, and you may lose what you have. This attitude often creates fear. Abundance is the attitude that with hard work and luck, you can have what you want. Note that this attitude focuses on possessions and rewards that may or may not completely fulfill you.

Prosperity is the ability to ride the waves of life, whether you experience wealth or poverty, and stay true to who you are. When you feel prosperous, the root chakra can withstand times of change, instability, and uncertainty. This attitude of prosperity cultivates trust, which is a key component of the root chakra.

Next time the root chakra gets fixated on survival and fluctuates between feelings of scarcity and abundance, focus on an attitude of prosperity. Trust that you are exactly where you need to be and trust in the wisdom of your soul.

Practice this powerful mantra to experience prosperity, penetrate the unknown without fear, and cultivate mental balance:

Aap Sahaaee Hoaa, Sachay Daa Sachay Dhoaa, Har, Har, Har

The divine has become my refuge. True is your support, great creative infinite energy

Relationship to Your Fears and Your Adrenal Glands

> Take a moment and think about the role fear plays in your life.
>
> *How often do you feel fearful?*
> *What are your main fears?*
> *Do your fears stop you from doing what you want?*
> *In what ways do your fears protect you?*

Fear is a natural emotion and a reaction to perceived danger. Its job is to keep you alive and safe. The main issue in the root chakra is fear. Staying alive, safe, secure, and stable are all elements of the root chakra. Fear is a tool to keep you safe. You need fear to know when to run, hide, and avoid dangerous situations. Fear can be a useful tool if used properly. Too much fear can stop you from taking risks, growing and expanding, forming meaningful relationships, and awakening the energy of the other chakras.

Fear is related to your fight, flight, or freeze response and triggers the adrenal glands to produce adrenaline to flee from danger, to fight it, or to freeze in place. This response helped our ancestors survive when a tiger was chasing them and their life was in danger. In today's society, many perceived threats trigger the fight, flight, or freeze response, even when we are not in actual danger. Overuse of the adrenal gland depletes your energy and weakens the root chakra. Because the adrenals sit on top of the kidneys, they are often linked together and both are associated with fear.

Rather than react to every fear that arises, cultivate a relationship with your fears and listen to them. Start by trying to differentiate between which fears are related to protecting your ego and which are responses to true dangers in your life.

Recognize these "Four Fatal Fears" and the role they play in your life[7]
Fear of failure
Fear of rejection
Fear of being wrong
Fear of emotional discomfort

---

7. Larry Wilson and Wilson Hirsch, *Play to Win: Choosing Growth Over Fear in Work and Life* (Austin, TX: Bard Press, 1998), 141–146.

These fears bombard your mind with images and situations of worst-case scenarios. Images of you being vulnerable, embarrassed, ashamed, humiliated, and eventually annihilated in some way. Your ego will try to avoid any situation in which you might fail, be rejected, be wrong, or be emotionally uncomfortable. If these fears go unchecked, the fearful mind takes over and you experience a constant state of fear, anxiety, and worry. Your energy will either be depleted or excessive in the root chakra.

Since the root chakra is your foundation, this energy imbalance will affect the health of all the other chakras. Cultivate a habit of communicating with your fears so you can befriend them and let them help you move forward in life.

Visualization to Befriend Your Fears

Take a moment and sit in a comfortable position. Close your eyes and visualize your fears knocking on your front door. Invite the fears in and sit with them in your living room, drinking tea together. Allow the fears to talk to you about all the dangers and pitfalls related to any risks you want to take, any changes you want to make, any ways in which you want to grow and expand.

Ask your fear, "From what are you trying to protect me?"

Listen deeply. Invite fear to go on a journey with you to connect with your other chakras. Take fear with you as you move into the second chakra and connect with your passions. Move into the third chakra and focus on your strengths. Move into the heart chakra with the fear and dwell in the love and compassion at your heart. Move into the fifth chakra and connect with your powerful ability to communicate and express yourself. Take fear with you to the sixth chakra and introduce fear to your soul, to your higher self, to the divine within you. Let fear talk to your wisdom and intuition. Reassure fear that you have many strengths and resources within you and in your life, which allow you to take risks and grow and expand. Thank the fear for protecting you.

Allow the fear to be your friend and your guide.

Questions

1. Which of these areas feels most balanced? Health, home, work, finances.
2. Which area has been most neglected?
3. In what ways can you give more attention and care to this area?
4. What are the incomplete projects in your life that may be draining your energy?
5. What will help you complete these projects?
6. What are your recurring fears?
7. How do these fears hold you back?

_____

_____

_____

_____

_____

_____

_____

_____

_____

_____

_____

_____

_____

_____

_____

Root Chakra Short Practice

Kicking the Floor

Lie down on the floor with knees bent and feet hip-distance apart. Alternately stomp the feet on the floor. Inhale through the nose and powerfully exhale through the mouth with a *ha* sound. Practice for one to three minutes.

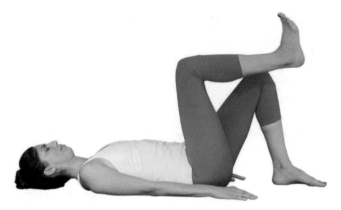

Benefits: Releases excess apana (energy of elimination) from the body and releases mental and emotional resistance to things you need to get done or move through.

Bridge Pose

Keep the knees bent with feet parallel and hip-distance apart. Keep the heels near the buttocks. Arms reach down to grab the ankles or rest on the floor with palms down. Inhale and push the feet down into the ground while lifting the thighs toward the ceiling. Walk the shoulder blades toward one another. Hold the pose with long, deep breathing and continue to lift a little higher with each inhalation. Practice for two to three minutes.

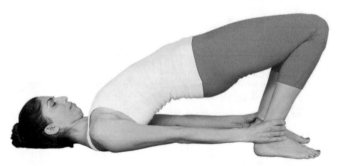

Benefits: Alleviates fear and anxiety, strengthens legs, stretches the thighs and abdominal area, and creates a deeper connection with the earth through the feet.

Tree Pose

Start in a standing position. Raise the right leg and place the sole of the foot along the inside of the upper thigh with the heel close to the groin and the toes pointing down. Bring the hands into prayer pose at the heart chakra. Keep lengthening the spine and push the foot and inner thigh toward one another. Keep the eyes open or closed. Breathe long and deep and connect with the earth qualities of feeling grounded, rooted, supported, nurtured, and strong. Switch sides.

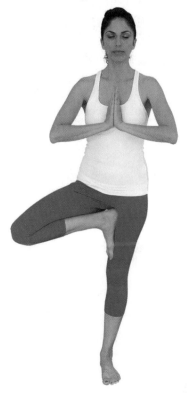

Benefits: Connects you to the nourishing energy of the earth and improves your balance.
Variation: Sole of the foot can rest against the ankle or calf instead of the inner thigh.

Mountain Pose

Stand with the feet together. Keep the shoulders down and the spine long. Keep the head balanced over the heart and the heart balanced over the belly button. Bring the hands into prayer pose. Breathe long and deep. Connect with your foundation, your roots, and the healing, grounding energy of Mother Earth.

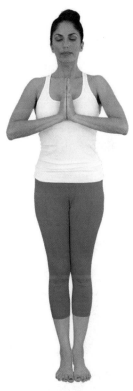

Benefits: Improves posture; strengthens thighs, knees, and ankles; and enhances body awareness.

Root Chakra Warm-Ups

Practice each pose for one to two minutes.

1. Left Nostril Breath

Sit in easy pose. Left hand rests on the knee in gyan mudra (thumb and index finger touching). Close off the right nostril with the right index finger and breathe long and deep through the left nostril.

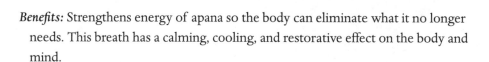

Benefits: Strengthens energy of apana so the body can eliminate what it no longer needs. This breath has a calming, cooling, and restorative effect on the body and mind.

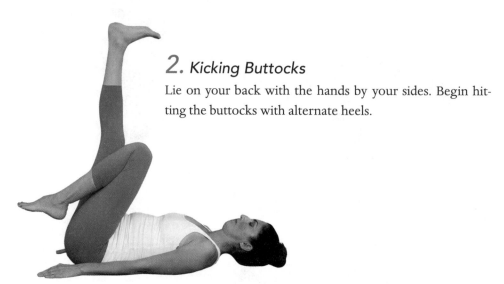

2. Kicking Buttocks

Lie on your back with the hands by your sides. Begin hitting the buttocks with alternate heels.

Benefits: Aids digestion and balances apana, the energy of elimination.

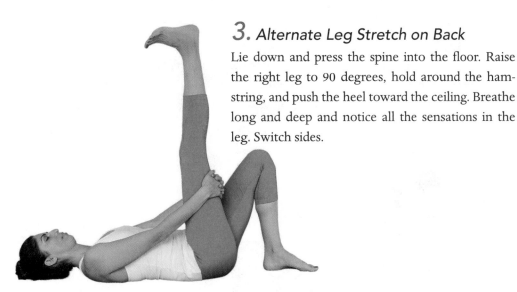

3. Alternate Leg Stretch on Back

Lie down and press the spine into the floor. Raise the right leg to 90 degrees, hold around the hamstring, and push the heel toward the ceiling. Breathe long and deep and notice all the sensations in the leg. Switch sides.

Benefits: Strengthens the muscles of the legs and stretches the hamstrings.

4. Bridge Pose Lifts

Hold on to your heels or keep your hands on the floor beside the hips. Push the feet and raise the thighs up, hold for a few seconds, and lower the hips back down. Continue at your own pace, inhaling up and exhaling down.

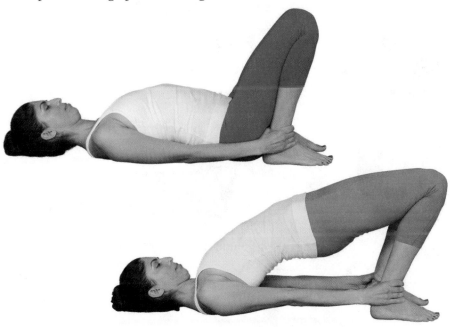

5. Cat Cow

Come onto all fours and place the wrists under the shoulders and the knees under the hips. Make sure there is space between the knees. Inhale and drop the spine down and lift the head up. Exhale and round the spine upward and drop the head down. Continue at your own pace.

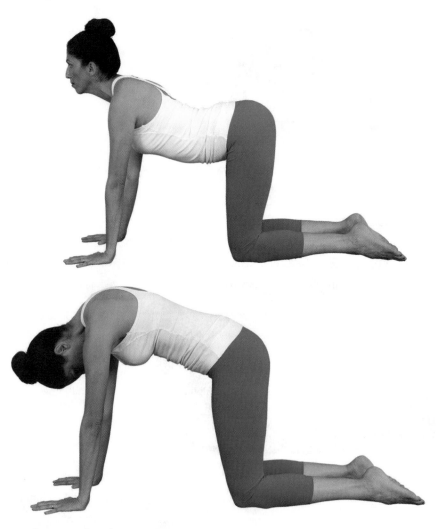

Benefits: Stretches the muscles along your back and neck, improves circulation, and balances the energy in all chakras.

6. Cow to Child's Pose

From cow pose, sit on the heels, forehead to the floor, and extend the arms forward. Inhale and return to cow pose. Exhale to child's pose and continue at your own pace.

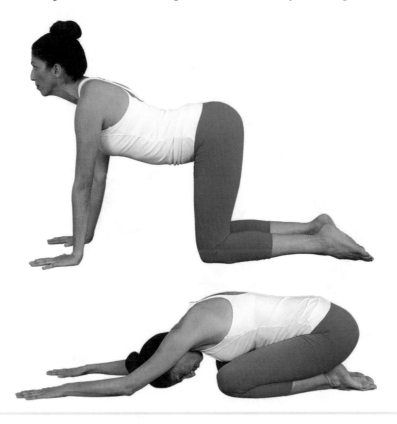

7. Triangle Pose

Begin in table pose with the wrists under the shoulders and hips over the knees. Push into the hands and feet and lift the body into a triangle. Lengthen the spine, draw the shoulder blades toward each other, relax the head, push the legs away from you, and press the heels toward the earth. Breathe long and deep.

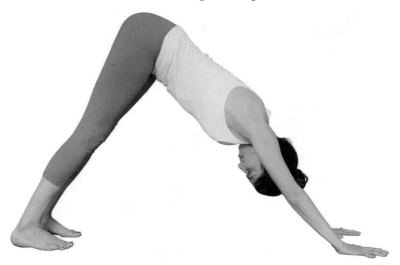

Kriya for Stability, Strength, and Endurance

This kriya is a strong physical workout that builds strength, flexibility, and endurance. This set promotes healthy digestion and elimination so the body can release what it no longer needs. A regular practice will help you stay grounded and steady under pressure.

Practice each exercise for one to three minutes unless otherwise specified.

1. Sit with the left heel on the perineum (the area between the sex organs and the buttocks) and the right leg extended straight out. If this is painful, you can rest the left foot against the inner right thigh. Bend forward and grasp the toes of the right foot. Breathe long and deep. Keep a light root lock applied, gently pulling up on the perineum, sex organs, and navel point. Switch sides.

To end: Inhale deeply and pull back on the toes. Completely exhale and apply a strong root lock.

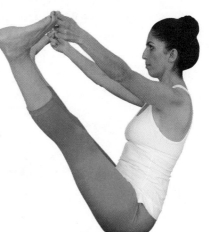

2. Bring the feet in front of you and interlace the middle and index fingers around the big toes. Keep the spine straight, engage the core, and straighten the legs out to 60 degrees. Gaze forward. Apply a gentle root lock.

Variation: Keep the knees bent and hold on to the toes, shins, or thighs.
To end: Inhale deeply, exhale, and apply a strong root lock.

3. Extend both legs straight out. Reach forward and hold on to the toes. Pull the spine up straight by pulling back on the toes. Pull the chin straight back. Begin long, deep breaths.
   Apply a strong neck lock.

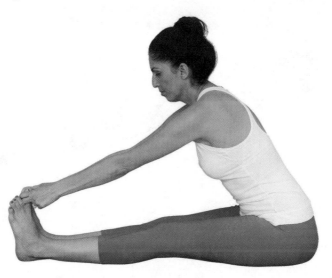

To end: Inhale, exhale, and apply a strong root lock.

4. Keep the legs extended straight, place the palms behind you, and lift the stomachand buttocks up until the body is straight, with only the heels and the palms on the ground. Bring the chin to the chest. Press the toes forward. Hold the posture with normal breathing.

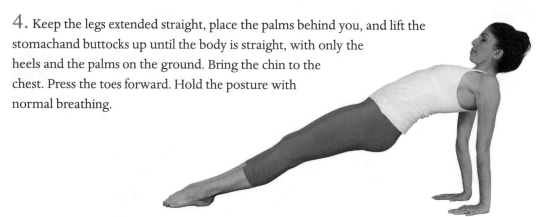

Variation: Keep the knees bent over the ankles and press up toward the ceiling.
To end: Inhale, exhale, and apply a strong root lock.

5. Lie on the stomach and put the palms on the ground under the shoulders. Inhale and slowly push off the ground with the body straight until you form a platform. Exhale as you slowly go down to the ground.

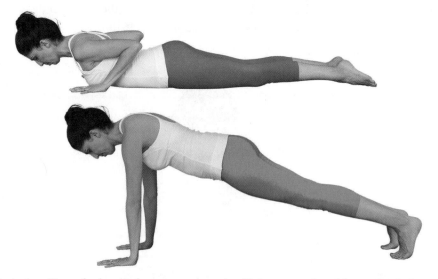

Variation: Keep the knees down as you push off the ground and lower back down.
To end: Inhale, exhale, and relax in child's pose for a few breaths.

6. Lie on your back. Place the elbows under the shoulders. Raise the buttocks up so the spine and body are straight. Chin is tucked in. Only the heels and elbows are on the ground. Press the toes forward. Breathe long and deep.

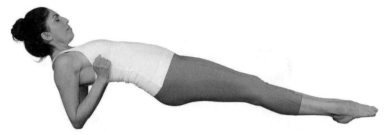

Variation: Keep the legs and buttocks on the floor and only lift the chest up.

To end: Inhale, then exhale completely and apply root lock.

7. Sit on your heels. Slowly lean back until the head and shoulders are on the ground. The arms are relaxed on the ground beside the legs. Keep a light, constant root lock applied.

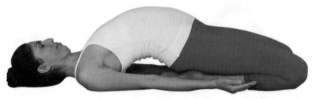

Variation: You can recline back on a bolster or a stack of blankets for additional support or keep your hands on the floor behind you and only recline as far back as is comfortable.

To end: Inhale, exhale, and apply a strong root lock.

8. Frog pose. Sit in a squatting position with the heels off the ground and touching. Fingertips are on the floor and the knees are out to the side. Head is in line with the spine. Inhale and push the hands into the floor and straighten the legs, bringing the head toward the knees. Quickly exhale and squat back down, making sure to keep the head in line with the spine.

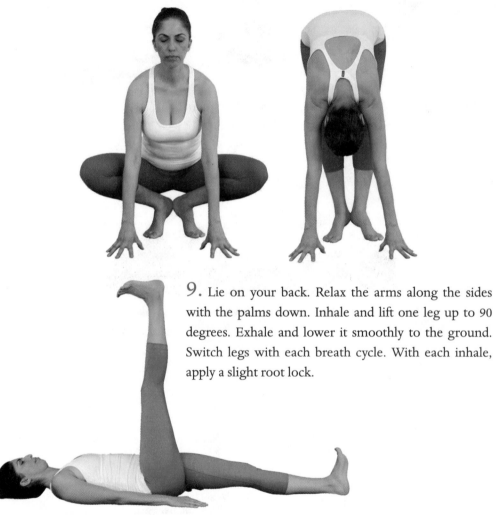

9. Lie on your back. Relax the arms along the sides with the palms down. Inhale and lift one leg up to 90 degrees. Exhale and lower it smoothly to the ground. Switch legs with each breath cycle. With each inhale, apply a slight root lock.

Benefits: Alternate leg lifts stimulate the energy of the lower intestines and circulate it throughout the entire navel area.

To end: Inhale, exhale, and relax for a few breaths.

10. Sit in a comfortable meditation posture. Pull in the navel point (area that is about two inches below the belly button) and apply root lock. Mentally scan your entire body. As you do this, your mind will have many thoughts. The thoughts will be related to the feelings and memories stored in different areas of the body. The subconscious mind will also release thoughts. Reject any thought that arises. Whether the thoughts are true or false doesn't matter.

Each thought naturally invites you to action or identification. Stay neutral. You are not body, mind, or spirit, but the consciousness that gives rise to and integrates all three. Continue for three to five minutes.

Relax for seven to ten minutes. Let the feet splay out to the sides. Relax the ankles, knees, hips, and entire spine. Soften the navel, chest, and shoulders. Relax the arms and fingers. Soften the throat, jaw, eyes, and top of the head. Surrender to the energy of the earth. Let the body sink more deeply into the floor, connecting you with your roots. In this peaceful space, visualize a beautiful red light showering you with healing and nourishing energy. Allow this spiraling energy of red light to fill you with strength, stability, and radiant health.

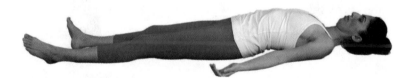

Meditation for Releasing Fear of the Future

This meditation helps you release fear and trust in the process of life. The crossed thumbs help neutralize the mind's anxious calculations to avoid fear and pain. This meditation will help you move forward in life and connect more deeply to your heart center and intuition.

Posture

Sit in easy pose.

Mudra

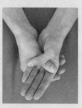

Place the back of the left hand in the palm of the right hand. The right thumb nestles in the palm of the left hand and the left thumb crosses it. The fingers of the right hand curve around the outside of the left hand and hold it gently. Holding your hands in this way will give you a peaceful, secure feeling. Place this mudra at your heart center with the palm-side resting against the chest.

Eye Focus

Eyes are closed and focused at the brow point.

Mantra

Listen to your favorite version of *Dhan Dhan Ram Das Gur.*

This mantra opens the heart to allow miracles to happen in all aspects of your life, including health, home, and finances.

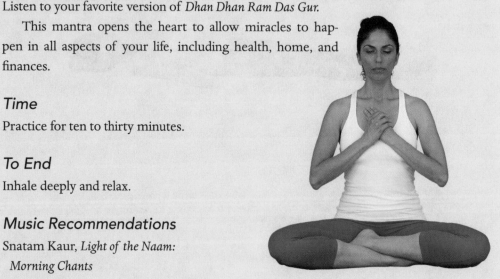

Time

Practice for ten to thirty minutes.

To End

Inhale deeply and relax.

Music Recommendations

Snatam Kaur, *Light of the Naam:
   Morning Chants*
Jai-Jagdeesh, *Miracles Abound*

Meditation for Prosperity

This meditation cultivates an attitude of prosperity. The mantra opens the mind and heart to attracting resources and opportunities that serve your highest good.

Posture

Sit in easy pose with a light neck lock.

Mudra

Arms are by your side, elbows slightly in, and the hands are in a straight line with the arms. Pull the arms slightly back to feel a stretch across the chest.

Eye Focus

Eyes are slightly open and focusing on the tip of the nose. Visualize green energy surrounding the hands and your entire body.

Mantra

Har Har Har (infinite creative energy)
Chant one Har per each second and pull the navel in. Let the breath regulate itself.

Time

Practice for ten to thirty minutes.

To End

Inhale, hold the breath, and connect with the grounding energy of your root chakra and the loving energy of your heart chakra. Relax.

Music Recommendations

Snatam Kaur, *Mantras for Prosperity*
Thomas Barquee, *Kundalini: Rise of the Soul*

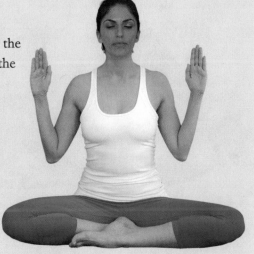

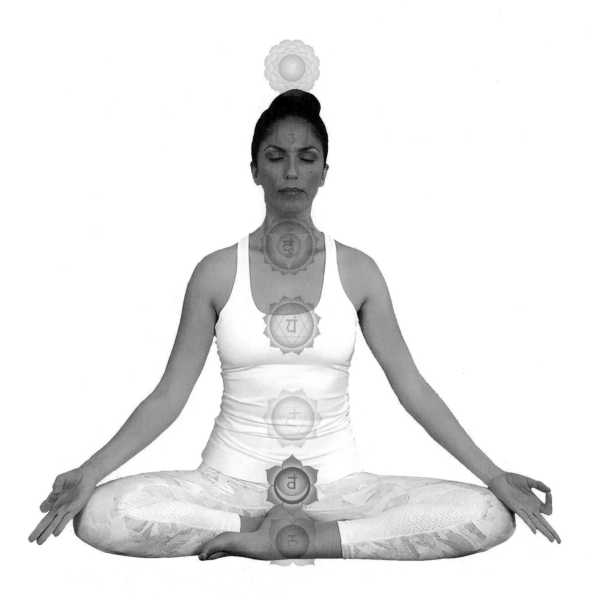

Explore your passion for life.

Chapter 3

SACRAL CHAKRA (2nd Chakra)

Sanskrit Name:	Svadhisthana (One's Own Place)
Main Issues:	Movement, desire, emotions, sexuality, and guilt
Element:	Water
Location:	Low back and sex organs
Color:	Orange
Goals:	Fluidity of movement, healthy connection to emotions, and ability to experience pleasure

Balanced Energy
- Graceful movements
- Ability to embrace change
- Emotional intelligence
- Nurturance of self and others
- Healthy boundaries
- Healthy enjoyment of sexual pleasure
- Passion for life

Deficient Energy
- Rigid
- Guarded
- Emotionally numb
- Lacking desire and passion
- Avoids pleasure
- Fears sexuality
- Fears change

Excessive Energy
- Overly emotional
- Seductive
- Self-indulgent
- Obsessive attachments
- Addictive personality
- Highly sexual
- Highly sensitive

Healing Practices
Spend time near water

Drink plenty of water

Psychotherapy to connect with or contain emotions

Enjoy healthy pleasures without guilt

Movement, dance, and yoga

Make rest a priority

Affirmations
I trust my feelings and give them ample room for self-expression.

I am more than enough.

I am open to receiving pleasure in my life.

I feel nourished and blessed.

I am excited about the possibilities in my life.

The Symbol

The symbol for the second chakra is a circle with six petals containing a silver crescent moon with the tips pointing upward. The two circles form the moon, which represents the water element, and water symbolizes emotional fluctuations, the ebb and flow of the tides, and change. The circles also refer to the cycles of birth, death, and rebirth. The six petals are associated with qualities that must be overcome to purify the sacral chakra—anger, jealousy, cruelty, hatred, pride, and desire.

Some versions of this symbol include a representation of an animal called a Makara, which is a type of fishlike crocodile that represents desire and sexual vitality. The seed sound at the center of this symbol is **Vam.**

Relationship to Water and Change

Take a moment to notice how you feel about change and movement.

*Do you flow with the changes in your life,
   or do you resist?*

*What's your relationship to water
   and how often do you spend time near water?*

What's your favorite type of physical movement?

How often do you practice this movement?

Water represents flow and movement. One of the goals of the second chakra is to get you moving. Movement creates change, growth, and expansion. The second chakra invites you to embrace change in your inner and outer world.

During times of change, chant the mantra *Sa Ta Na Ma*. It means infinity, life, death, and rebirth. This mantra is a reminder that change is a natural part of life, and all things move through this cycle. There is a beginning, middle, and end to everything. The more you allow and surrender to this process of change, the more relaxed and at peace you can be during times of change and transition.

From the solidity of the earth, we move to the ebb and flow of chakra two and the water element. Water moves, flows, follows the path of least resistance, and creates change.

Relationship to Health and Nourishment

Notice if your lifestyle makes room for rest, nourishment, and balance.

How do you release stress and tension from your body?
What signals do you look for to let you know you've exceeded your boundaries or limitations?
How do you recharge your energy?
What nourishes you?

Humans are wired to be alert and on the lookout for dangerous situations in order to survive. This programming makes it challenging for us to relax and let go. We have to intentionally cultivate the habit of nurturing ourselves, slowing down, and relaxing.

If you stay in the first chakra mindset, you remain focused on surviving and working. You ignore your body's need to rest, relax, and take time off for pleasurable and enjoyable activities. To restore health to the second chakra, find a balance between "doing" and "being." Figure out what drives you to keep doing. What are you striving for? What do you long for that you can't get enough of? Feeling like you are not enough is often the underlying cause of continually doing and accomplishing.

The second chakra heals when you understand that you are enough and what you do is enough. Learn to say no when you are overworking yourself or others are taking advantage of you. Honor your body and your energy and use these resources wisely.

Take time to give yourself a daily rest, plan activities that are fun and enjoyable, get enough sleep, and set clear boundaries with yourself and others.

Make a list of things you need and want to feel healthy and nourished. Notice if you neglect your needs or your wants. How often do you let yourself indulge? Be mindful that all our needs and wants are different, and truly listen to your own guidance over what others think you should want or need.

Needs: Eight hours of sleep, one cup of coffee, journal in the mornings, eat warm cooked veggies and rice, exercise daily with yoga or long walks, meditate daily

Wants: Sleep in, two or more cups of coffee, go on a weekend retreat, eat pizza, exercise every other day, meditate when I feel like it

Relationship with Pleasure

Consider what brings you pleasure in your life.

How much of your day is spent taking care of your needs versus your wants?

How often do you allow yourself to experience pleasure in your life?

What do you desire?

In the second chakra, you move beyond your needs and into the realm of pleasure and desire. Your wants are connected with what brings you pleasure.

When the second chakra is balanced, you are excited and passionate about life. You allow yourself enough time for relaxation, pleasure, and enjoyment. Life feels colorful and fun. Pleasure is experienced through the senses and invites the outer world in.

Make a list of your top ten pleasures and find ways to weave them into your daily routine.

My Top 10 List:

1. Meditate
2. Play badminton
3. Hang out at a coffee shop
4. Eat a sweet pastry
5. Go for a walk in the woods with my husband

6. Watch an episode of *The Golden Girls*

7. Get a massage

8. Give Bodhi (my dog) a belly rub

9. Dance

10. Daydream about traveling the world

Relationship to Emotions

Emotions are a form of energy that manifest in the body through sensation. They want to be felt, heard, experienced, and released.

What can you notice in your relationship with your emotions?

What is your relationship with your 6 Core Emotions: happiness, sadness, fear, anger, surprise, and disgust?*

Do you take time to process your emotions?

What emotions are you uncomfortable feeling and expressing?

* Paul Eckman, "Universal Emotions," https://www.paulekman.com/universal-emotions/.

Emotions can largely be seen as a reaction to pain or pleasure. When you experience pain, you shut down, and when you experience pleasure, you expand. You have a choice to feel and express emotions or suppress and numb them. Often our relationship to emotions is learned from our family dynamics. As children, you may have been taught to feel and express your emotions, told to suppress them, or made to feel guilty and ashamed for feeling or expressing your emotions.

As adults, we may either overidentify with our emotions or underidentify with them. Healing the sacral chakra requires a balanced approach to experiencing our feelings. The first step is to identify the sensations associated with the emotion and then to create space between you and the emotion and engage in a process of inquiry.

Next time a strong emotion arises, be curious about the experience and see what you discover. Ask yourself the following:

- What is this emotion trying to tell me about this experience or situation?
- In what way is this emotion trying to protect me?
- Have I experienced this before?
- Am I reacting to something in this moment, or am I being triggered by a past event? What's unresolved for me about that past event?

Emotional work is the process of recovering lost feelings, bringing them to life again, and resolving them. This may require the help of a trusted friend or a good therapist. If the first chakra is strong and grounded, you will be more comfortable feeling emotions and moving toward growth and expansion without feeling like you are losing yourself. It may help to write down your feelings.

Which feelings do you embrace, and which do you avoid?

Jealousy, sadness, anger, envy, joy, disgust, pride, irritation, embarrassment, frustration, courage, tension, fear, love, stress, empathy.

You can't heal what you don't feel.

Relationship with Duality

Take a moment to notice the dualities at play in your life.

What are you attracted to that is different from you?

How do you honor the masculine and feminine energies within you?

What helps you move out of your comfort zone and connect with new people and experiences?

In the second chakra, you move into the realm of duality, expansion, and choice. You want to experience something or someone different from yourself. You have a desire to merge with another, to move into other states of consciousness, and grow.

Duality brings the concept of polarity: male and female, light and dark, up and down, good and bad, pleasure and pain. A goal of the second chakra is to hold the tension of opposites without forcing one or the other. You can be both sad and happy. You are both feminine and masculine. A balanced second chakra is able to see the whole and embrace the polarities within.

Relationship to Sexuality

In the second chakra, our attention shifts to include others and how they can bring more pleasure into our lives.

What are your values and attitudes toward sexuality and sensuality?

Are you comfortable asking for what you want in your primary relationships?

Do you set clear boundaries in your relationships?

The second chakra moves you toward other people and lights up when you feel a connection with others. You are attracted to those who you believe will bring more pleasure and excitement into your life. The attraction to others in the second chakra also ignites our sexual urges and desires. Our ultimate desire is to experience sexuality through the senses and merge with another to experience intimacy. Intimacy requires a genuine connection, honest communication, and respect for one another's feelings.

Relationship with Guilt

Notice how often you feel guilty in your life.

What is your relationship with guilt and how often do you experience it?

What sensations do you experience when feeling guilty?

What helps you alleviate guilt?

Guilt is a strong emotion that most of us learn in early childhood. The purpose of guilt is to let you know when you have done something wrong and have gone against your own values. Guilt helps you understand how your behavior impacts others and prompts you to reexamine your own behavior. Healthy guilt serves to help you stay aligned with your moral compass. Unhealthy guilt makes you feel bad for things that aren't harming anyone and deprives you of pleasure and enjoyment.

Healing the second chakra requires understanding the difference between healthy and unhealthy guilt. Healthy guilt can be a helpful inner guide for staying true to your own values and taking responsibility for your actions. Unhealthy guilt stops the flow of pleasure, blocks your passions, and suppresses your feelings. Unhealthy guilt says you shouldn't need anything and you shouldn't feel a certain way: "I shouldn't feel this way and I shouldn't want that." Next time guilt arises, ask yourself, "Is this feeling trying to teach me something helpful about my behavior or is it an irrational response to this situation?" Notice when guilt arises, communicate with it, and respond from a place of awareness rather than from a habitual reaction.

Remember to ask if the guilt you feel is a learned behavior from your family or from your own feelings. Remind yourself to make this distinction in order to transform the guilt into acceptance. Pleasure may have been taboo in your family, and beliefs about denying yourself pleasure might be at play in your subconscious mind. What are your beliefs about pleasure, joy, and relaxation? Are you ready to transform these beliefs?

Relationship to Your Feminine and Masculine Energy

Notice your relationship to being and doing, to giving and receiving, and to feeling and thinking.

How do you connect with your feminine and masculine energies?
Does one dominate or are they balanced?
Are you more drawn to the sun or to the moon?

Divine feminine energy is the goddess energy within. All of us, regardless of gender, have both feminine and masculine energy within us. The second chakra represents feminine energy in the form of emotions, receptivity, giving, relaxing, creating, and nurturing. The third chakra represents masculine energy and action, vitality, and focus. We need both energies to live a full and balanced life.

The moon represents feminine energy and the sun, masculine energy. The left side of the body relates to the feminine and issues related to our mothers, and the right side relates to the masculine and issues with our father. Notice if you have more issues on the right or left side of your body.

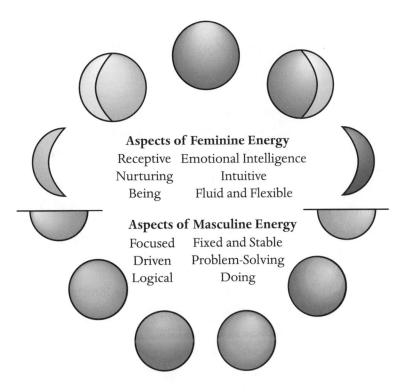

Aspects of Feminine Energy

Receptive   Emotional Intelligence
Nurturing   Intuitive
Being   Fluid and Flexible

Aspects of Masculine Energy

Focused   Fixed and Stable
Driven   Problem-Solving
Logical   Doing

Mantra to Awaken the Feminine Energy

Adi Shakti, Adi Shakti, Adi Shakti, Namo Namo

Sarb Shakti, Sarb Shakti, Sarb Shakti, Namo Namo

Pritham Bhagvati, Pritham Bhagvati, Pritham Bhagvati, Namo Namo Kundalini Mata Shakti,
Mata Shakti, Namo Namo

I bow to the primal power

I bow to the all-encompassing power and energy

I bow to that which God creates

I bow to the creative power of the Kundalini, the Divine Mother Power

This devotional mantra invokes the primary creative power, which is manifest as the feminine. It calls upon the mother energy. It will help you be free of insecurities that block you from moving forward.

Music: Nirinjan Kaur, *From Within,* and Ajeet Kaur, *Shuniya*

Feeling Your Feelings

I used to dread being asked, "What are you feeling?" I'd stare back at the person with a blank look on my face and feel absolutely nothing. I'd do my best to change the subject or leave the conversation. In my childhood home, no one asked me how I was feeling. I internalized everything and kept it in. When I did express my feelings, I was often judged and ridiculed because my feelings differed from those of my family.

I didn't realize until I was an adult that much of the pain and tension in my body were from repressing my feelings. When I began journaling, I discovered that writing about my feelings was a safe place to start exploring this realm. I started to recognize what anger and sadness felt like in my body, and I began to learn a new vocabulary to communicate my emotions.

While journaling, I realized that I attracted people into my life who were open with their emotions and very communicative about their needs and wants. I started to pay attention to these people and learn from them rather than resent them for doing something I couldn't. I recognized them as teachers helping me grow my skills in this area.

In my meditation practice, I became more aware of my emotions and gave them the time and space to be expressed, including letting myself cry when tears welled up. The more I let myself feel, the lighter I felt in my body. My emotions wanted to be acknowledged. If I dealt with them on a daily basis in my meditation and journaling practice, they didn't overwhelm or scare me.

Once I cultivated a relationship with my emotions, my health, energy, and vitality returned. For some people, feeling their emotions and expressing them feel like the most natural thing in the world. Most likely they learned this beautiful quality from their parents. The rest of us had to learn as adults to feel and express. It's like learning to ride a bike as an adult—it's possible, but it takes time and patience and can feel quite awkward at times.

Questions

1. What excites you and ignites your passions?

2. How much do you physically move during the day? How can you invite more movement into your life?

3. Where do you resist movement and change in your life (job, relationship, health)?

4. How comfortable are you expressing your emotions and withholding emotional expression when necessary?

5. Do you feel emotionally satisfied with your life?

6. What do you long for?

_____

_____

_____

_____

_____

_____

_____

_____

_____

_____

_____

_____

_____

_____

Sacral Chakra Short Practice

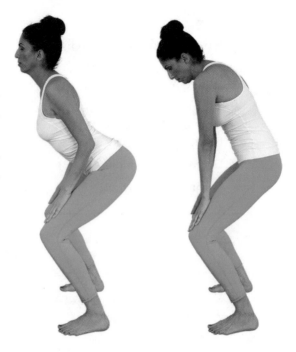

Standing Pelvic Tilts

Stand with the feet hip-distance apart and hands on top of the thighs. Inhale, bend the knees, and extend the spine forward. Keep the knees bent, exhale, and push the spine back. Continue back and forth at your own pace for one to two minutes.

Benefits: Releases tension and stress in the pelvic area and brings balance to the second chakra.

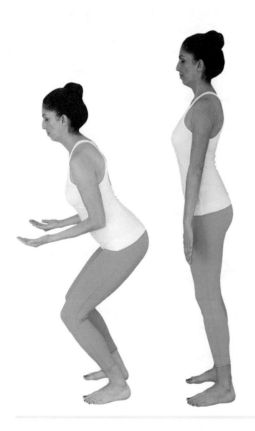

Standing Pelvic Thrusts

Stand with the feet hip-distance apart. Inhale and bend the knees as if you were going to sit in a chair, with the forearms parallel with the floor and palms up. Exhale through the open mouth with the sound *ha* and straighten the legs while keeping the knees soft and lowering the arms by your sides.

Benefits: Releases tension and stress in the pelvic area and brings more balance.

Dancing

Move the body to music that is fun and uplifting. Move the hips, legs, spine, shoulders, and head. Get uninhibited and move the energy in the body. Get out of your head and into your body as you move rhythmically to your favorite music. Continue for at least five minutes.

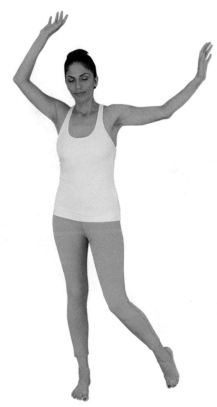

Benefits: Releases tension in the body, creates more ease and flow, and brings joy and relaxation to the second chakra.

Sacral Chakra Warm-Ups

Practice each pose for one to two minutes.

1. Pelvic Tilts

On your back, bend the knees and place your feet hip-width apart. Move the hips and low back off the floor on the inhale and press down into the floor on the exhale.

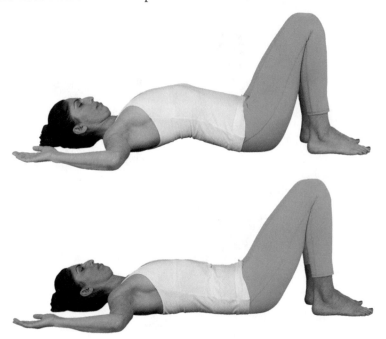

2. Spinal Pulse

On your back with knees bent, start to slide the spine up and down without lifting it off the floor. Push into the feet and slide the spine toward the head and then back down toward the feet.

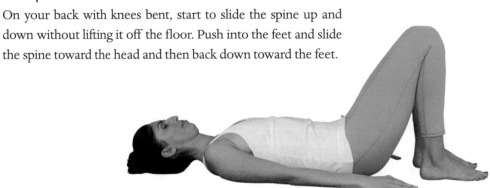

3. Cat Stretches

Lie on your back and bring the right knee to your chest. Drop the knee over to the left side while keeping the shoulders on the floor. Inhale, return to center, and repeat on the other side. Keep your head neutral or turn toward the direction you are stretching. Continue alternating side to side.

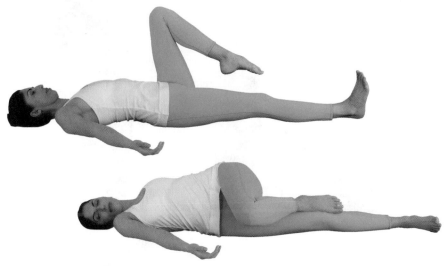

4. Eye of the Needle

On your back, bend both knees and lift your right foot and place it over the left thigh, making the number 4 shape. Lift the left knee toward your chest and wrap the hands around the left hamstring. Hold with long, deep breaths as you press the right knee away from you and the left knee toward you. Switch sides.

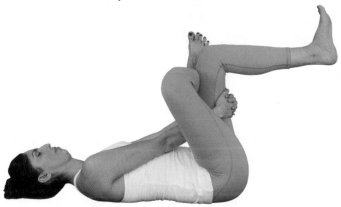

5. Cat Cow

Come onto all fours and place the wrists under the shoulders and the knees under the hips. Make sure there is space between the knees. Inhale and drop the spine down and lift the head up. Exhale and round the spine upward and drop the head down. Continue at your own pace.

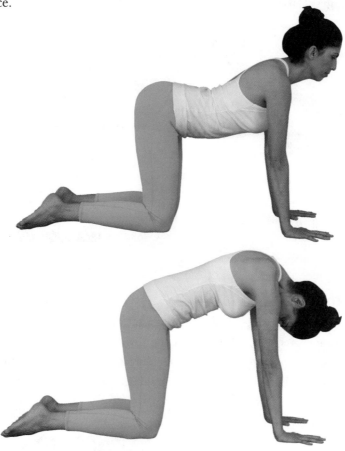

6. Locust Lifts

Lie on the stomach and extend the arms forward with palms touching. Inhale and lift the arms and legs as high as you can and breathe long and deep.

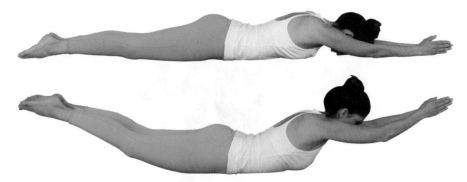

Benefits: Massages the kidneys and strengthens the entire back.

7. Child's Pose to High Cobra

Sit on the heels and stretch the arms forward in a child's pose. Spread the fingers wide and bring the head up. Keep the hands and arms where they are. Come up onto the knees and then push up with the hands into a high cobra with the shoulders away from the ears. Exhale and push back into child's pose. Continue alternating between the two poses. Inhale forward and exhale back.

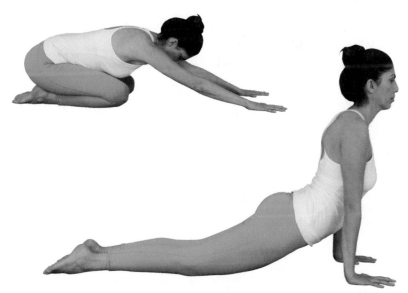

8. Child's Pose with Wide Knees

Push back into child's pose with the knees as wide as your mat. Arms rest in front. Sink into the hips and deepen the breath.

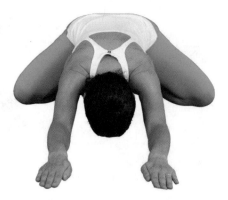

9. Pigeon Pose

Begin in table pose with the arms under the shoulders and the knees under the hips. Cross your left foot in front of the right knee. Slide and lengthen your right leg straight back. You can use a blanket under the hips if needed. Inhale and lengthen your spine, exhale and lower your chest toward the floor. If the head does not reach the floor, you can rest it on the forearms or a blanket. To come out of the pose, slowly push your spine up, uncross your legs, and switch sides.

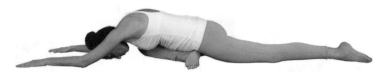

Benefits: Opens the hips, aligns the pelvis, stretches the thighs, hip flexors, and hip rotators. Increases circulation to the pelvic floor.

Sat Kriya Workout

This set will energize and balance the lower triangle. Sat Kriya strengthens the entire sexual system and stimulates the flow of energy in all the chakras. This set helps relax phobias about sexuality. It allows you to control sexual impulses by rechanneling sexual energy into creative and healing activities in the body. General physical health is improved since all the internal organs receive a gentle rhythmic massage from this exercise.

1. Sat Kriya

Sit on the heels with the arms overhead and the palms together. Interlace the fingers except for the index fingers, which point straight up. To connect with your masculine energy, cross the right thumb over the left, and to connect with your feminine energy, cross the left thumb over the right. Begin chanting *Sat Nam*. Powerfully chant *Sat* and pull the navel back toward the spine. Chant *Nam* as you relax and release the navel. The breath will take care of itself. Chant at a moderate pace. Continue for one to three minutes.

> *To end:* Inhale, exhale, and apply root lock. Relax on your back for one to three minutes.

2. Sat Kriya

Repeat Sat Kriya for one to three minutes and then relax for one to three minutes.

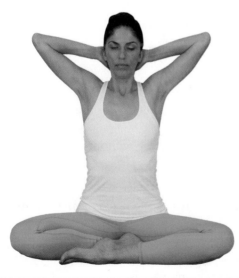

3. Chest Stretch

Sit in easy pose with an erect spine. Interlace the fingers and place the palms at the back of the neck. Spread the elbows open so they point away from the sides of the torso. Concentrate at the brow point. Breathe long, deep breaths. Continue for one to three minutes. Then inhale and hold the breath briefly and exhale.

4. Sat Kriya

Repeat Sat Kriya for one to three minutes and then relax for one to three minutes.

5. Frog Pose

Squat down into frog pose with the heels together and lifted. Keep the heels in this position throughout the exercise. Inhale as the buttocks goes up and the head goes down toward the knees. Exhale as you return to the squat position with the head up. The fingertips stay on the ground in front of the feet throughout the motion. Repeat twenty-five times. Relax for one minute.

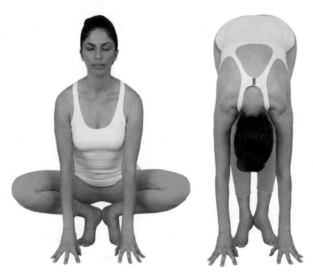

Variation: Use a block instead of the floor to rest the fingertips.

6. Sat Kriya

Repeat Sat Kriya for one to three minutes and relax for one minute.

7. Frog Pose

Practice ten times. Take a few breaths and begin the next posture without much rest.

8. Sat Kriya

Repeat Sat Kriya for one to three minutes. Take a few breaths and begin the next posture without much rest.

9. Frog Pose

Practice fifteen times. Take a few breaths and begin the next posture without much rest.

10. Sat Kriya

Repeat Sat Kriya for one to three minutes. Take a few breaths and begin the next posture without much rest.

11. Frog Pose

Practice ten times. Take a few breaths and begin the next posture without much rest.

12. Sat Kriya

Practice Sat Kriya for three to five minutes.

> *To end:* Inhale deeply and hold with root lock for thirty seconds. Then exhale completely and hold the breath out with mahabandha (great lock) for as long as comfortable. Repeat this breath holding cycle two more times.

Relax *for seven to ten minutes*

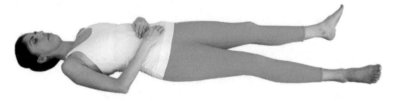

Rest on your back with the legs straight and the feet splayed out to the sides. You can place a bolster or blanket under the knees for additional support. Make sure you are warm and comfortable as you begin this relaxation. Relax the feet and let them splay out to the sides. Soften the ankles, calves, and shins. Let the thighs melt into the floor. Visualize a beautiful, spiraling, orange light around the hips and sex organs, restoring balance to your second chakra. Allow your breath to find its own natural rhythm while softening the navel area. Let the spine sink into the earth. Relax the chest, shoulders, arms, and hands. Soften the muscles in the neck and throat. Let your entire face soften. Visualize a beautiful orange light showering you with healing energy and restoring your passion for life.

Meditation for the Sacral Chakra

This meditation brings healing energy to ailments of the second chakra.

Posture

Sit in easy pose with your spine straight. Apply neck lock.

Mudra

The hands are chest-width or slightly wider and at a 45-degree angle toward the earth. Elbows are raised. The fingers of each hand are together and the thumbs point up. The arms from the elbows to the hands are stiff. Move the arms sharply down; the hands move toward each other, four to six inches apart, in a single stroke, with the beat of the music, approximately one movement per second. Arms return to the original position with each stroke. As your hands move inward, tighten the sex organ and release it as the hands move back to the starting position.

For men, the tightening is centered at the base of the sex organ. For women, the contraction includes the clitoris. This is not a root lock—the anus and navel point are not contracted with the sex organ.

Breath

Breathe naturally.

Eye Focus

The eyes are focused at the tip of the nose.

Mantra

Listen to the mantra *Ek Ong Kar Sat Gur Prasad* (the creator and creation are one).

Time

Practice for ten to thirty minutes.

To End

Inhale, hold the breath, and tighten every muscle in the body. Hold for fifteen seconds and relax. Repeat the cycle two more times.

Music Recommendation

Jai-Jagdeesh, *Expand into Intuitive Knowing*

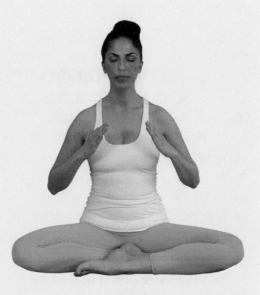

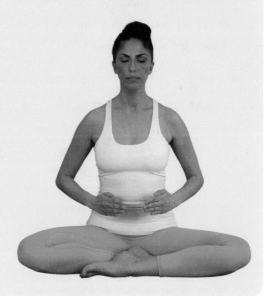

Meditation for Emotional Balance

Practice this meditation when you feel emotional upheaval and distress. The mantra helps activate relaxation, self-healing, emotional relief, and inner peace.

Posture

Sit in easy pose and apply a light neck lock.

Mudra

The hands rest on the knees, palms up and elbows straight. Choose the mudra that most resonates with you in this moment.

Feminine energy: Left hand, the thumb and middle finger touch. Right hand, the thumb and ring finger touch.

Masculine energy: Left hand, the thumb and ring finger touch. Right hand, the thumb and middle finger touch.

Eye Focus

Keep the eyes slightly open.

Mantra

Guru Guru (the teacher that brings one from darkness to light)
Wahe Guru (the experience of ecstasy)
Guru Ram Das Guru (the wisdom that comes from the infinite)
Chant in a soft monotone voice. Each repetition takes about eight to ten seconds.

Breath

Inhale between each repetition.

Time

Practice for ten to thirty minutes.

To End

Inhale, exhale, and relax.

Music Recommendation

Sat Purkh, *The Guru Within*

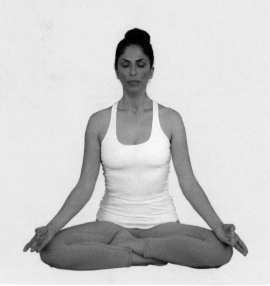

Ignite your energy and vitality.

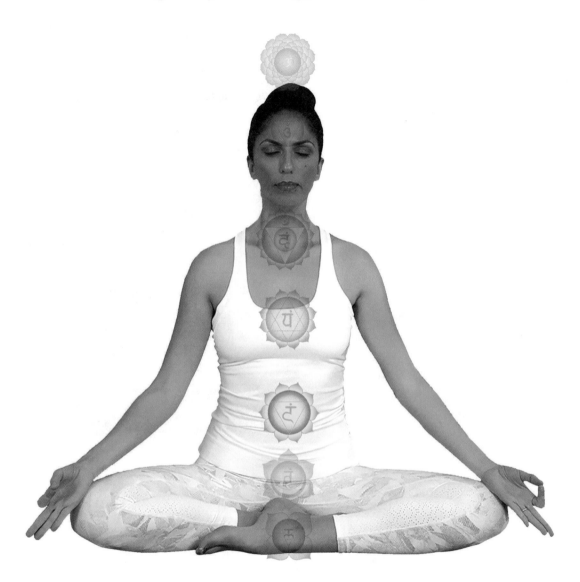

Chapter 4

NAVEL CHAKRA (3rd Chakra)

Sanskrit Name: Manipura (Lustrous Gem)

Main Issues: Energy, power, will, ego, anger, and shame

Element: Fire

Location: Solar plexus, stomach, intestines, liver, and pancreas

Color: Yellow

Goals: To act, to achieve, and to build confidence

Balanced Energy
- Proactive
- Reliable and responsible
- Resilient
- Healthy self-esteem
- Able to achieve goals
- Confident
- Spontaneous
- Good sense of humor

Deficient Energy
- Passive
- Blaming
- Low energy
- Low self-esteem
- Tendency to be cold
- Attracted to stimulants
- Lacking self-discipline
- Poor digestion

Excessive Energy
- Dominating
- Controlling
- Hyperactive
- Driven compulsively
- Tendency to be hot
- Attracted to sedatives
- Arrogant
- Stubborn

Healing Practices

Vigorous exercise

Risk-taking

Stress management and relaxation exercises

Psychotherapy to manage issues around anger and shame

Engage in non-goal-oriented activities

Laugh, play, and connect with the inner child

Affirmations

I am resilient.

I act with courage and strength.

I am confident and powerful.

I accept responsibility for all my decisions.

I follow through on my commitments.

I am playful and see the humor in life.

The Symbol

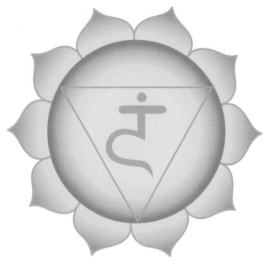

The third chakra symbol is a circle with ten petals forming a lotus with a downward-pointing triangle inside the circle. Some depictions show ten petals inscribed with da, dha, na, ta, tha, da, dha, na, pa, and pha, representing spiritual ignorance, thirst, jealousy, treachery, shame, fear, disgust, delusion, foolishness, and sadness. Inside the lotus is a downward-pointing triangle, which represents the fire element and suggests the movement of downward-flowing energy.

In some versions of this symbol, there is a ram inside the lotus. The ram is an animal of power, and the seed sound symbol is **Ram.**

Relationship to Fire

Notice your relationship with the fire fuels the energy for metabolism, confidence, courage, motivation, and creativity.

How often do you feel uncomfortably hot or cold?
What qualities do you associate with fire?
How do you feel near the sun or near a fire?

The fire element is necessary for change and transformation. In the body, fire is essential to transform food into energy, ingesting what the body needs and eliminating what it doesn't. On a mental and emotional level, the fire element helps you process ideas and moves you into action.

The fire element conveys heat, sharpness, brightness, and upward-moving energy. When the fire element is balanced, you feel naturally joyful, generous, and enthusiastic. Your digestion and elimination are regular and easy. Insufficient fire can leave you feeling cold, depressed, and lethargic. Excess fire can leave you feeling hot and agitated and, if left unchecked, can burn out of control and manifest as uncontrolled anger.

Relationship with Digestive System

Notice how different foods affect your energy and mood.

How would you describe the health of your digestive system?

Which foods make you feel lethargic, bloated, and uncomfortable?

Which foods make you feel energized, light, and focused?

Do you slow down at mealtimes?

The digestive system is the group of organs that break down food in order to absorb its nutrients. The nutrients are used by the body as fuel to keep all the systems working. The leftover parts of food that cannot be broken down, digested, or absorbed are excreted as bowel movements. The digestive tract forms one long tube through the body from the mouth to the anus.

The health of your digestive system affects your energy, mood, feelings, and thought processes. Your ability to digest food impacts how well you function in your life. Kundalini Yoga helps keep your digestive system healthy by increasing the secretions of gastric juices and digestive enzymes that speed up a sluggish metabolism and increase fire energy at the navel point, which aids digestion. Yoga also increases the body's ability to eliminate. Upper arm exercises stimulate meridian points corresponding to the stomach and colon.

Mindful Eating Practices

Incorporate these practices for one meal a day or a few days a week and notice any shifts in your energy and your digestion:

- Drink a glass of room-temperature water thirty minutes before you eat.
- Eat your meal in a peaceful place.
- Pause for a minute to express gratitude for your meal and for all the people involved in getting it to your table.
- Connect with your senses as you eat.
- Put your utensil down after each bite.
- Chew your food thoroughly.
- Relax for a few minutes after your meal.

Relationship with the Ego

Notice your relationship to your ego, which represents your individuality, sense of self, and self-esteem.

What defines who you are?

Are you content with who you are and what you do?

Do you feel confident and comfortable applying your strengths to move forward in life?

When was the last time you took a risk?

What risks are you avoiding?

Ego identity is related to your sense of self and self-worth. A healthy ego gives you a strong sense of self and the confidence to commit to your goals and take risks. A weak ego is inconsistent, indecisive, and fearful of confrontation. An overdeveloped ego is manipulative, exploitive, and inflated. Overcoming challenges and taking thoughtful risks builds confidence and resiliency, which lead to a healthy and balanced ego.

Yogis strive to cultivate a healthy ego that is aligned with a higher purpose in order to grow and expand in awareness and consciousness. Without this connection to a higher purpose or calling, the ego stays limited in scope and serves only its own needs, which are insatiable; the ego always wants more money, awards, possessions, recognition, and accolades. A spiritual practice, especially meditation, continually chisels at the ego to move beyond false identifications and continual self-references. First you cultivate a strong, healthy ego, and then you train it to align with a higher purpose and serve the greater good.

Relationship to Willpower and Commitment

Willpower is your ability to focus and direct your energy toward a specific goal to influence an outcome.

How often do you use your willpower?
How often do you follow through on your commitments?
What distracts you from completing goals?

The quality of your life depends on the actions you take. Notice your relationship with your willpower and your ability to create change and transformation in your life. To reclaim the power of your will, realize that everything you do is a choice. Even the act of not choosing is a choice. Shift your thinking from *I have to* to *I choose to*, so that every action in your life is a choice. Feel empowered by this simple shift in thinking and look at your life from a different perspective.

Willpower is needed to move through difficult, challenging, and unpleasant tasks in order to achieve our goals and dreams. If the third chakra is weak, we give up when things get hard, and the energy gets stuck at the navel point. Willpower is like a muscle that gets stronger when used and weaker when ignored. Start with achieving small tasks to build strength in this muscle. Visualize your energy, power, and strength as bigger than the challenge you are facing. Focus on your strengths and own your own power.

Research shows that we are born with one third of our strengths, and the rest we learn over our lifetime.[8] This is great news because we can leverage the strengths we were born with and cultivate new strengths that help us become stronger and more resilient.

Take a moment and make a list of your inner strengths and visualize all the ways in which these strengths have helped you overcome adversity in the past. Now visualize how these strengths can help you move forward in life and experience victory.

See if any of these inner strengths resonate with you: calm, peaceful, enthusiastic, curious, content, creative, courageous, loving, generous, resilient, focused, fun, strong, open-minded, motivated, intuitive, organized, humorous, witty, charming, and so on.

8. Rick Hanson, *Hardwiring Happiness: The New Brain Science of Contentment, Calm, and Confidence* (New York: Harmony Books, 2013), 4–6.

Another way to strengthen the navel chakra is to make lists. Research shows that when you write lists, you are much more likely to achieve the items on the list (and handwriting is considerably more effective than typing). An effective practice for strengthening your focus and willpower is to handwrite a daily list. When you wake up, decide on the five most important items you need to accomplish and do them first. Make sure your list is specific, and that you have the time and resources to accomplish everything you've listed. When I cross an item off my list, I feel a boost in energy and a readiness to tackle the next item.

On a bigger scale, writing down your goals can motivate and inspire you to achieve them. Make a list of ten goals you want to accomplish this year. Write your goals in the present tense. For example, "I speak fluent Spanish." Or, "I meditate for thirty minutes every day." Review your list and choose the one goal that would have the greatest positive impact on your life. Then write it on a separate sheet of paper and break down the goal into projects and tasks. Projects related to your goal would take months to accomplish and tasks involve daily items. Then do something every day to move closer to the goal.

Relationship to Anger

Notice your relationship to anger.

How often do you experience anger?
Do you express or repress your anger?
How do you respond to anger directed at you?

Anger is an emotion that arises to protect you from injustice, pain, and frustration. Without anger, you wouldn't have the energy to protect and defend yourself. However, most of us rarely learn how to harness this energy and use it wisely. Many people repress anger, which creates stress and tension in the body, or they express it inappropriately in ways that are hurtful and damaging.

What should you do with anger? Bring consciousness and awareness to your anger. Let go of any judgments about the anger arising—we cannot control what arises in us, only how we react to it. Recognize the sensations that come up when you are getting angry. Then pause and take a few deep breaths. Ask the anger, "What are you protecting me from?" and wait to hear the answer. Connect with your body and the sensations in your body when you listen for the answer. Your health and well-being suffer when you repress or inappropriately express your anger.

Tips to Manage Your Anger

- Exercise vigorously.
- Start a meditation practice and commit to it for at least forty days.
- Take breaks during the day to check in with your emotions, especially during stressful days.
- When anger arises, breathe deeply, and create distance between yourself and your anger. Move into the role of observer/witness and rise above the details and specifics of the situation, see the big picture, and then act from this place of awareness.
- When you are calm, express your anger or frustration using "I" statements and avoid blame or judgment.
- Take a break from junk food and alcohol to give your liver a rest, as the liver is said to energetically store anger.

Cool Off Your Anger with Sitali Breath

This breathing exercise delivers power, strength, and vitality. It can have a cooling and cleansing effect on anger. Initially, the tongue tastes bitter, and will eventually become sweet.

Sit in a comfortable position. Roll the tongue into a *U*, with the tip just outside the lips. Inhale deeply through the rolled tongue. Bring the tongue back in, close the mouth, and exhale through the nose. If your tongue doesn't roll, bend the sides of the tongue as much as possible.

Continue for three minutes in the evening. Practice for longer periods to experience a deep meditation and bring healing energy to your body and digestive system.

Relationship with Shame

Notice the role shame plays in your life.

How often do you feel shame?
What triggers shame?
How do you deal with shame when it comes up?

Shame is the feeling that something is wrong with you. Shame develops from these types of messages in childhood:

- "What is the matter with you?"
- "You never do it right."
- "You don't have what it takes."
- "You're not as good as everybody else."

If you hear these messages repeatedly, they become internalized and affect your self-worth. These messages can deplete the third chakra, causing us to become afraid of confrontation and risk-taking, or they can create excessive energy in the third chakra, leading to compulsion and a need to assert power over others. Feelings of shame can make us feel isolated and lonely, but it's important to remember that all humans experience this emotion, and the feeling will pass.

One way to heal shame is to focus on the overall purpose of your actions rather than on receiving acknowledgment from others. Shame is a powerful emotion to confront and elevate. You confront the shame by discrediting the negative thoughts that say something is wrong with you. Those thoughts are not true and are from your past. As a child, you had no choice but to listen to them. As an adult, you can take back your power and discredit the self-defeating and negative thoughts. You eliminate the shame by recognizing your self-worth and valuing your presence rather than your achievements.

To elevate the shame, try this Loving Kindness Meditation to Melt Away Shame: Mentally say the following phrases for several minutes to adopt a friendlier and kinder attitude toward yourself when feelings of shame envelop you. Replace judgment with kindness. Either mentally repeat these phrases for a few minutes or write them down. Notice what comes up as you practice this. It may take time to work through resistance that arises when you are creating a new habit. You are welcome to create your own phrases if these don't resonate with you.

May I be Safe.
May I be Healthy.
May I be Happy.
May I be Peaceful.
May I be Loved.
May I be Accepted.
May I Live with Ease.

Meditation to Build Confidence

Practice this meditation for three minutes to build self-esteem and confidence and to overcome feelings of shame.

Sit in easy pose, with a straight spine. Place your hands in a meditative mudra of your choice. Look at the center of your chin through closed eyes, or focus at the tip of your nose with your eyes a tenth open.

Inhale deeply, suspend the breath, and mentally recite,

I am Bountiful. I am Blissful. I am Beautiful.

Exhale completely and hold the breath out as you mentally recite,

Excel. Excel. Fearless.

Questions

1. What gives you energy and what drains it?
2. What do you consider to be your greatest achievement?
3. How often do you let yourself play, laugh, and let go of achievement?
4. How do you handle conflict in your life? Is your strategy effective?
5. How often do you feel in control of your day? How often do you use your willpower?

_____

_____

_____

_____

_____

_____

_____

_____

Navel Chakra Short Practice

Sufi Grind

Sit in easy pose and hold on to your knees. Move the hips and waist to the left, making a big circle around with the spine. As you move, feel the stretch in the ribs and heart chakra. Continue for one minute with long, deep breaths, and then reverse the direction.

Benefits: Strengthens the digestive center, processes energy at the navel point, and balances the fire element.

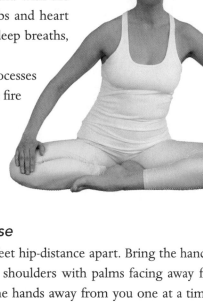

Power Pose

Stand with feet hip-distance apart. Bring the hands in front of the shoulders with palms facing away from you. Push the hands away from you one at a time as you also stomp the ground one foot at a time. Make it a powerful movement and chant *ha* as you move the hands and feet powerfully. Continue for one to three minutes.

Benefits: Connects you with your energy, strength, and power. Helps you feel victorious.

Wood Chopper

Stand with the feet apart. Inhale and interlace the fingers and bring the arms overhead. Then bend the knees and swing the arms down and between your legs as you exhale through the open mouth and make the sound *ha*. This breath is healing for the lower triangle of chakras and releases energy. Visualize chopping wood and breaking through the challenges in your life. Continue for one to three minutes.

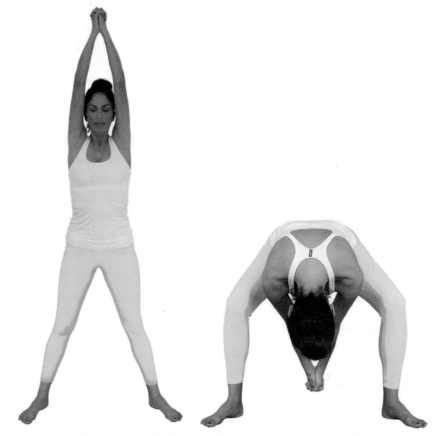

Benefits: Strengthens the third chakra, releases pent up energy, and energizes your system.

Shake to Your Favorite Music

Stand up and shake your body. Shake the arms, shoulders, spine, hips, legs, feet, and head. This is not dancing, but vigorous shaking to create a sweat. Continue for three to five minutes.

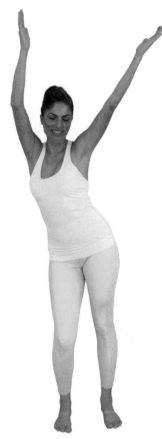

Benefits: Improves circulation, distributes the energy, sweats out toxins, and
  burns fat.

Navel Chakra Warm-Ups

Practice each pose for one to two minutes.

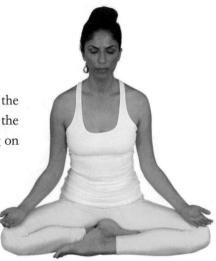

1. Breath of Fire

Sit in easy pose and begin breath of fire. Allow the breath to be rapid, continuous, and equal on the inhale and exhale. Palms are open and resting on the knees.

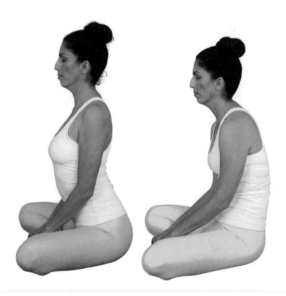

2. Spinal Flex

Sit in easy pose with the hands holding the shins. Keep the shoulders over the hips. Inhale, extend the spine forward, and exhale, push the spine back.

3. Spinal Twist

Bring the hands to the shoulders with the fingers in front and the thumbs in back. Inhale and twist to the left and exhale and twist to the right. The head, shoulders, and waist move together in a smooth motion. Keep the elbows up at shoulder height.

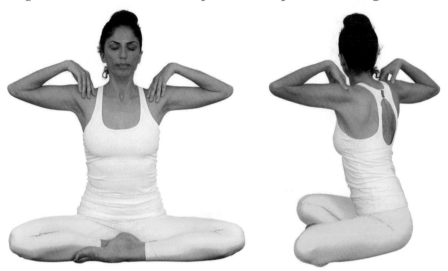

4. Cat Cow with Kicks

Come onto all fours. Inhale and drop the spine down as the head moves up toward the ceiling. Extend the right leg as far back as possible. Exhale and bring the head and knee toward each other while engaging the abdominal muscles. Continue for one minute and then switch sides.

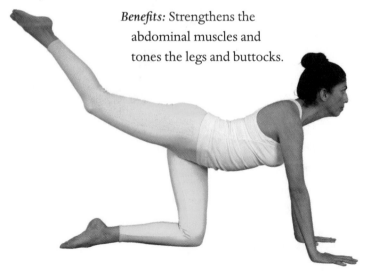

Benefits: Strengthens the abdominal muscles and tones the legs and buttocks.

5. Triangle Pose to Cobra

Lie on your stomach with your hands under your shoulders. Push up into a high cobra with the hips off the floor. Exhale, engage the core, and push the body into triangle pose. Continue to flow between the two poses with the breath.

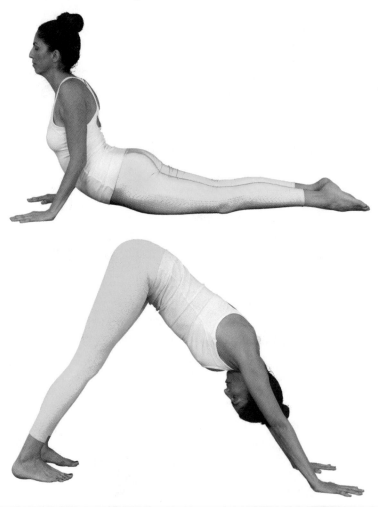

6. Standing Side Bends

Come to standing. Interlace the index fingers and stretch to the left side on the inhale and to the right side on the exhale. Move from the hips and feel the stretch in your ribs. Continue side to side.

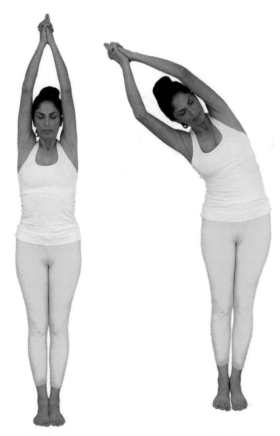

Benefits: Lengthens the abdominal muscles and hips while improving flexibility of the spine.

7. Archer Pose Variation

Stand with the feet as wide as possible. Turn the right foot to a right angle and bend the knee until it is over the ankle. Bring the arms out to the sides and bend the back elbow. Keep the front arm extended. Curl the fingers of both hands and stretch the thumbs up. Bend and straighten the front leg while chanting *Har*, which means infinite creative energy. Eyes are open and focused at the tip of the extended thumb, which represents the ego. Continue for one to two minutes, and then switch sides.

Benefits: Generates fearlessness and balances and strengthens the nervous system.

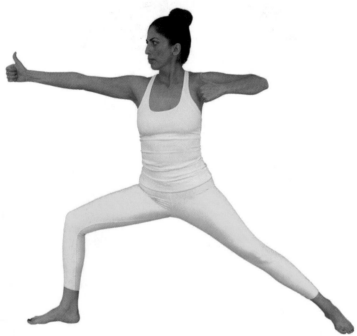

8. Forearm Plank

Lie on the stomach with elbows under the shoulders and the palms together. Curl the toes under and lift the body up into a straight line and hold. Engage the core muscles and lift the shoulder blades toward the ceiling.

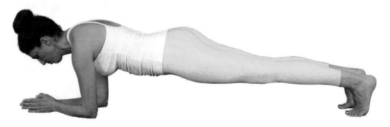

Kriya for Abdominal Strengthening

This kriya gives you a strong physical workout. It strengthens the navel point, abdominal muscles, and lower back. It improves circulation and strengthens the nervous system so that you can handle the challenges of life. It also helps strengthen the digestive system.

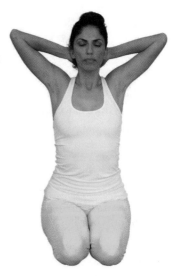

1. Sit on the heels or in easy pose. Interlock the fingers behind the neck in venus lock. Spread the elbows wide apart. Perform breath of fire for two minutes.

> *Variation:* Sit on a block or blanket if you experience any pain in your knees or ankles or sit in easy pose.
>
> *To end:* Inhale, hold the breath, exhale, and relax.

2. Lie on the stomach. Reach back and grab the ankles. Pull the ankles toward the buttocks while keeping the chest on the ground. Hold for two minutes with long, deep breathing.

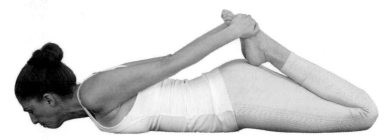

> *To end:* Inhale, hold the breath, exhale, and relax.
> *Benefits:* Healing for the digestive system.

3. Stretch pose. Lie on the back and raise the head and heels six inches off the ground. Keep the low back pressed into the floor and engage the abdominal muscles. Keep the chest lifted and the back of the neck long. Eyes are open and looking at the toes. Place the hands by the thighs with fingers pointing toward your feet. Begin breath of fire and hold the pose for two minutes.

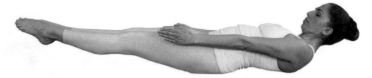

Variation: You can raise the legs higher to keep the low back pressed on the floor or keep the knees bent.

To end: Inhale, hold and engage all your muscles, exhale, and relax for a few breaths.

Benefits: Adjusts and strengthens the navel point, tunes up your nervous and digestive systems, and strengthens the reproductive organs and glands.

4. Lie on your back and lift the legs twelve inches off the floor. Bring your right knee into your chest as you extend the left leg out. Switch sides, continuing the push-pull movement for two minutes.

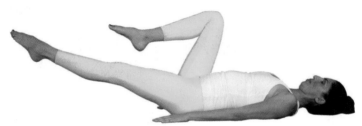

To end: Inhale, hold the legs up, exhale, and relax.

5. Still on your back, keep the legs together with the toes pointed forward, and raise both legs to 90 degrees on the inhale. Exhale and lower them down. Keep the lower back pressed into the floor as you move the legs up and down. Keep the chin down and the neck relaxed. Continue for two minutes.

Variation: Raise and lower one leg at a time.

To end: Raise both legs to 90 degrees, take a deep inhale, hold, and as you exhale, lower the legs down. Relax. Hug the knees into your chest if you feel any discomfort in your lower back.

6. Lie on the stomach. Place the palms on the ground under the shoulders and slowly lift the spine up, but keep the hips on the floor. The arms are either straight or with a slight bend in the elbows. Press the hands forward as you draw the elbows back. Lift the feet up toward the head. Hold for two minutes.

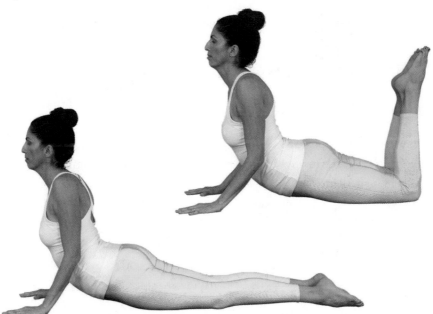

Variation: Keep the forearms on the floor and lift the spine up. You can also keep the legs on the floor.

To end: Inhale, hold and arch the spine up, exhale, and slowly lower your body down. Relax.

7. Still on your back, bring both knees to your chest and hold on to your shins or the backs of the knees and start to roll forward and back on your spine. Continue for two minutes.

> *To end:* Rock yourself up to sitting and take a deep breath.
>
> *Benefits:* Massages the organs and spine and distributes the energy throughout the body.

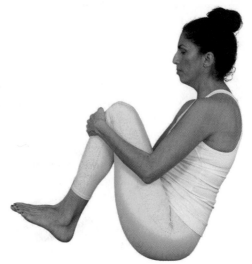

8. Locust pose. Lie on your stomach. Extend the arms forward with the palms flat together. Arch the back so that the arms, chest, and legs lift off the ground. Hold this extended locust pose with breath of fire for two minutes.

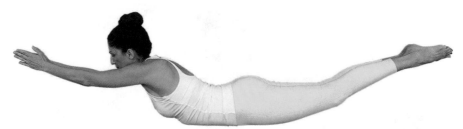

> *To end:* Inhale, hold the pose, lift a little higher, exhale, and relax.
>
> *Benefits:* Strengthens the lower back and hamstrings, tones the abdominal muscles, and increases circulation.

9. Bow pose. Still on the stomach, bring the feet toward the buttocks and reach back and grab the ankles. Push the feet into the hands to engage the muscles in your legs. Press the shoulder blades together. Continue to hold for two minutes with breath of fire.

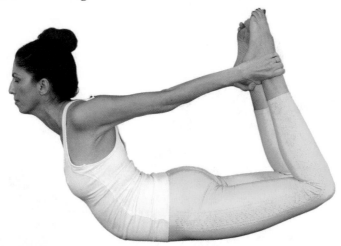

Variation: Let go of the ankles and stretch the arms and legs toward each other while keeping the chest lifted.

To end: Inhale, hold, exhale, and slowly lower yourself down and rest on a cheek or your chin for a minute.

Benefits: Strengthens your back, arms, and buttocks, massages your organs, and opens the shoulders and heart chakra.

10. Side stretch. Stand up and keep the legs together. Extend the arms to the sides, parallel to the ground, with palms facing down. Without twisting the torso, bend to the left with a deep inhale and bend to the right with the exhale. Continue this metronome motion for two minutes.

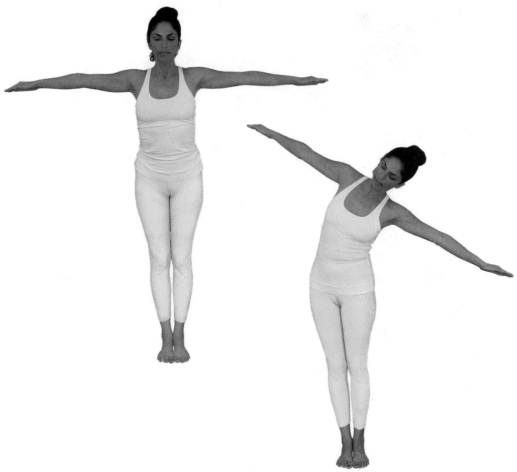

To end: Inhale, come to center, and exhale.

11. Still standing, spread the legs about two feet apart. Bring the arms out to the sides, parallel to the floor. Inhale and stretch the left arm back parallel to the ground as the right hand comes to the heart chakra; exhale as the right arm stretches back parallel to the ground and the left hand comes to the heart chakra. Continue alternating from side to side for two minutes.

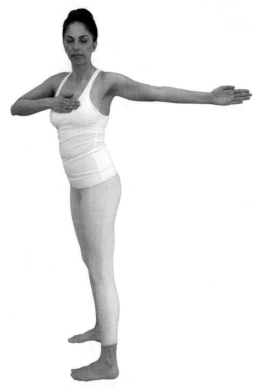

To end: Inhale, bring both hands to the heart center, and exhale.

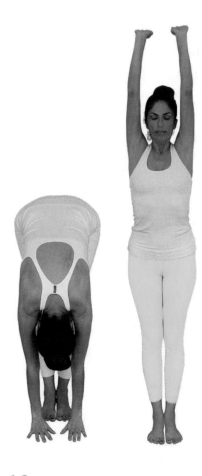

12. Still standing, raise both arms straight up with palms facing the ceiling. Exhale as you bend forward from the hips and either touch the palms or the fingers to the ground. Inhale, push into the feet, lift up the body, and stretch the hands toward the ceiling. Continue for two minutes.

To end: Inhale, stretch the arms up, exhale, and relax.

Benefits: Stretches the entire spine and reduces fatigue and tension.

13. Lie on the back. Repeat exercise 4 for two minutes. Keeping the legs parallel, bring your right knee into your chest as you extend the left leg out. Switch sides, continuing the push-pull movement. Breathe deeply.

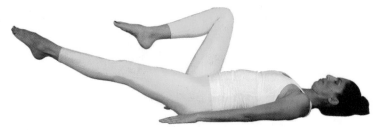

To end: Inhale, hold the legs up, exhale, and relax.

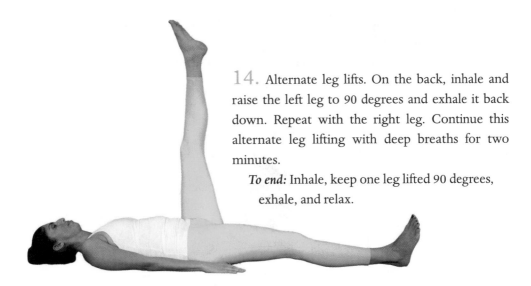

14. Alternate leg lifts. On the back, inhale and raise the left leg to 90 degrees and exhale it back down. Repeat with the right leg. Continue this alternate leg lifting with deep breaths for two minutes.

To end: Inhale, keep one leg lifted 90 degrees, exhale, and relax.

15. Seated boat pose. Sit with both legs extended out. Engage your core and keep the chest lifted. Raise the legs 60 degrees from the ground and extend the arms parallel to the floor with the palms down. Begin breath of fire. Continue for one to two minutes.

Variation: Keep the knees bent and hold on to the thighs, or keep one leg on the floor and one leg lifted.

To end: Inhale, hold, and exhale. Relax.

Benefits: Strengthens the core, optimizes circulation to the digestive system, and helps develop focus.

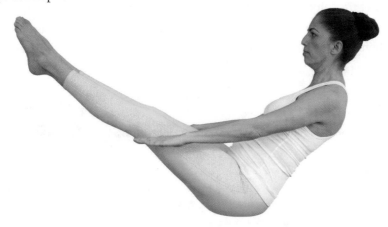

16. Sat Kriya with palms in prayer pose above the head. Sit on the heels with the arms stretched up and the palms together. Pull in the navel point in as you chant *Sat* and relax the navel point as you chant *Nam*. Continue rhythmically for two minutes.

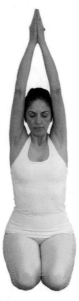

To end: Inhale deeply, hold the breath, apply root lock, and relax.

Relax for seven to eleven minutes. Rest on your back with the legs straight and the feet splayed out to the sides. Make sure you are warm and comfortable as you begin this relaxation. Soften the ankles, calves, and shins. Let the thighs melt into the floor. Visualize a beautiful, spiraling, yellow light around the belly button, restoring your energy, vitality, and light. Allow your breath to find its own natural rhythm while softening the navel area. Let the spine sink into the earth. Relax the chest, shoulders, arms, and hands. Soften the muscles in the neck and throat. Let your entire face soften. Visualize a beautiful yellow light showering you with healing energy and awakening your inner sun.

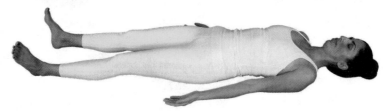

Meditation to Connect with Your Source of Infinite Energy

This meditation will connect you with your inner source of energy and strength. Practice this meditation when you feel disconnected from your own power and vitality.

Posture

Sit in easy pose.

Mudra

Stretch your left arm out to the side with the fingers in gyan mudra and the palm up. The right elbow is bent, the palm faces forward, and the hand is at the level of the ear. The right thumb and sun finger (ring finger) connect to form surya mudra while the other fingers point upward.

Eye Focus

Eyes are closed.

Breath

Inhale and exhale. Hold the breath out and pull in the navel, mentally chanting *Har* with each pull of the navel. Begin by chanting *Har* eight times with the breath held out. When you are comfortable with that, increase the number of times you pull the navel in and mentally chant *Har* sixteen times.

Mantra

Har (infinite creative energy)

Time

Start with three minutes and build up to ten minutes.

To End

Rapidly pump the navel as many times as you can, either with the breath held in or with the breath held out.

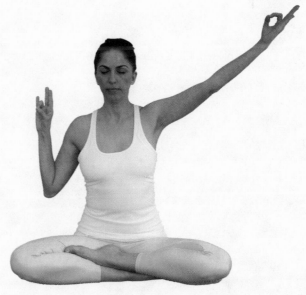

Meditation to Release Inner Anger

Practice this meditation for forty days to transform your relationship with anger and experience new levels of peace and acceptance within yourself.

Posture

Sit in easy pose with a straight spine and a light neck lock.

Mudra

Arms are stretched out straight to the sides. There is no bend in the elbows. The Jupiter (index) finger points upward and the thumb locks down the other fingers. The Jupiter finger, representing knowledge and expansion, should be kept stiff and straight during the meditation.

Eye Focus

The eyes are closed. Concentrate on your spine.

Breath

Inhale deeply through the rolled tongue (sitali breath) and exhale through the nose.

Mantra

There is no mantra with this meditation.

Time

Start with three minutes and build up to ten minutes.

To End

Bring the hands to your heart center and sit for a few minutes, noticing what you notice.

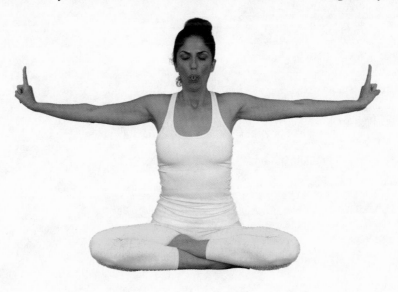

Part 3
The Gateway

The fourth chakra is known as the gateway between Earth and heaven and the balance point between the lower and higher chakras. When the fourth chakra is balanced, we experience deep levels of love, compassion, and forgiveness toward ourselves and others. We experience giving and receiving and finding balance in all aspects of life in this chakra.

Our consciousness moves beyond our own needs and desires, and we want to help and serve others in genuine and meaningful ways. We are even willing to make sacrifices in order to help others. We transcend from a place of "me" to a place of "we." Our consciousness expands to encompass the well-being of others as well as ourselves. We see ourselves as part of a collective and empathize with the global community. The energy of the fourth chakra inspires us to serve the greatest good in ourselves and others.

The fourth chakra needs a strong and balanced lower triangle to fully open, thrive, and experience genuine love.

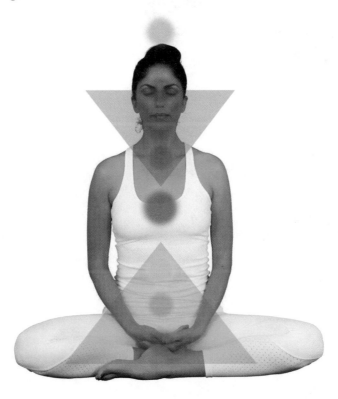

Dwell in unconditional love.

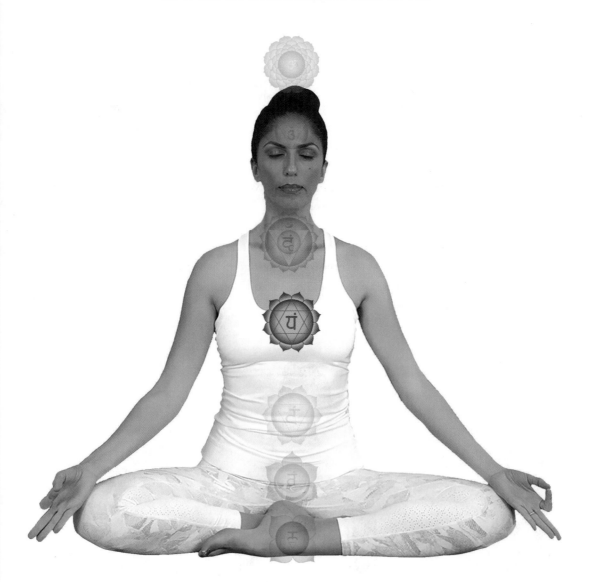

Chapter 5
HEART CHAKRA (4th Chakra)

Sanskrit Name: Anahata (Unstruck Sound)

Main Issues: Love, relationships, balance, service, and grief

Element: Air

Location: Center of chest and between shoulder blades

Color: Green

Goals: To love, to be compassionate, and to serve

Balanced Energy

- Compassionate
- Empathetic
- Accepting
- Self-loving
- Peaceful
- Centered
- Forgiving

Deficient Energy

- Withdrawn
- Antisocial
- Excessive boundaries
- Critical
- Intolerant
- Fear of intimacy
- Lack of empathy

Excessive Energy

- Clingy
- Possessive
- Poor boundaries
- Codependent
- Lacking in discrimination
- People-pleasing
- Need for attention and approval

Healing Practices

Movement with the arms

Cultivate self-love and acceptance

Forgive the past, including those who hurt you

List all the things, people, and experiences you love and fill your heart with gratitude

Watch inspiring movies

Volunteer

Affirmations

I love who I am and all that I do.

I see myself and others with love.

I give and receive with an open heart.

I am grateful for all the relationships in my life.

I am in balance with life.

My heart is overflowing with love and joy.

The Symbol

The symbol of the fourth chakra is a lotus with twelve petals that contain two overlapping triangles, creating a hexagram. These triangles represent the energy of the higher and lower chakras coming together at the heart chakra to create balance and integration. The downward-pointing triangle signifies the lower nature of humans and is connected to the earth energies, and the upper triangle represents the higher nature and is linked to our spiritual energies. The masculine principle of Shiva and the feminine principle of Shakti meet at the heart chakra to create union.

The twelve petals of the heart chakra represent the twelve mental modifications—hope, anxiety, endeavor, possessiveness, arrogance, incompetence, discrimination, egoism, lustfulness, fraudulence, indecision, and repentance.

Below the heart chakra is a smaller center called the Ananda Kanda, translated as the space of bliss, made up of a circle with eight petals. Contained within the circle is the tree of life and an alter decorated with precious jewels. It is said that our true self resides here surrounded by unconditional love. Meditating on the Ananda Kanda can grant us our deepest wishes.

Some versions of this symbol include an antelope, a gentle, horned creature that runs in the wild with tenderness and grace. The seed mantra of the heart chakra is **Yam.**

Relationship to the Air and Your Breath

Take a moment and notice your breathing and the sensations around your chest, shoulders, and neck.

Are your breaths full and deep or shallow and erratic?

Do you ever find yourself holding your breath?

How often do you think about your breathing in your daily life?

Air represents the breath of life and influences your energy, mood, and mental focus. The element of air represents expansiveness and movement. On a physical level, it relates to the quantity and quality of your breathing. The inhale delivers oxygen to the lungs and blood, while the exhale releases carbon dioxide from the tissues of the body. On an energetic level, the inhale brings in life-giving energy known as prana, and the exhale releases the energy of elimination known as apana. The balance of prana and apana in the body determines your energy level, vitality, and overall health and well-being.

The relationship with your breath is the foundation of any yoga practice. First, connect with the breath in your yoga and meditation practice, and then maintain that connection throughout your day. When you feel stressed and overwhelmed, take a deep breath through your nose and exhale through the open mouth. Let it go. When you feel tired and mentally drained, take deep breaths through the nose, expanding the body on the inhale, and lengthening the spine on the exhale.

Some yogis believe that at birth we are given a specific number of breaths, and when we reach that number, we expire. In order to live a long, healthy life, slow down the breath.

Relationship to Love and Self-Compassion

> Take a moment and visualize the people, places, things, and experiences you love.
>
> *What does love feel like in your body when you are with these people, places, things, and experiences?*
>
> *What makes you feel loved?*
>
> *How do you express love to others?*
>
> *In what ways can you be kinder to yourself?*

The heart chakra thrives on feelings of love, compassion, and connection. Self-compassion is creating a supportive, kind, and encouraging relationship with yourself.

The heart chakra is called the gateway between the needs of the ego—related to the lower chakras—and the spiritual connection of the higher chakras. We can feel love in the lower chakras, but that kind of love comes attached with strings and conditions. The love at the heart chakra is unconditional and connects you to universal love so that we feel love for others outside of our family, friends, and community.

When the heart chakra opens, we understand that we are part of humanity, able to see beyond our immediate environment, and we feel a connection with all beings. The shift from the lower chakras to the heart chakra is transformational because the ego learns to move beyond its own needs and transcends fear to experience love. Being in the heart chakra opens us to serving the greater good.

As the heart chakra opens to others and the world, it also opens more deeply and lovingly toward the self in the form of self-compassion. When the heart chakra is open and balanced, you practice kindness toward yourself instead of judgment and criticism. Self-compassion allows us to see our failures and inadequacies as part of the human experience and provides a safe and caring space for us to grow and learn from that experience. Self-compassion does not mean we get a pass from responsibility and accountability in life. It means that when we fall and fail, we are the supportive coach who helps us up with kindness and love rather than the critical coach who belittles us with criticism and shame. Which coach would you rather have in your life?

Self-Compassion Daily Break

A few times a day, bring your hand to the center of your chest, take a few deep breaths, and intentionally send yourself a kind thought. If you can't think of anything, recall the last time a friend said something kind to you and focus on the sensations that this memory evokes in your body. Stay with this thought for twenty seconds to a minute, breathe deeply, and connect with the sensations in your body. It's normal for this exercise to feel awkward, but it's worth the short-term discomfort to cultivate a more loving and supportive relationship with yourself in the long run.

Relationship to Your Shadow and Authentic Self

Bring your awareness to the relationships in your life.

How well do your friends know you?

What aspects of yourself do you share with the world and what aspects do you hide?

In your childhood, were there certain behaviors you were rewarded for and other behaviors you were punished for?

Do you remember the form of the reward and the punishment?

How would you describe your authentic self?

Your authentic self is who you are at your core. It is the part of you that isn't defined by your job or status. It is all the things that are uniquely yours and resonate with you on a deep level rather than what you believe you are supposed to be.

From a young age, we receive programming from the world about what people love in us and what they reject. Because we desire and crave love, we repeat the behaviors that bring us love and suppress the behaviors that provoke rejection. Over time, we create personas that accentuate the way we are supposed to behave in different social situations.

Unconditional love requires us to accept all aspects of our being. To heal the heart chakra, we need to recognize the aspects of ourselves that we rejected or suppressed and bring them to light. The more we can accept who we are, and not who we think we should be, the more accepting and compassionate we can be with others. When we show up being ourselves, we create more meaningful connections with others and create more peace in our lives. Opening up to yourself and others takes time and practice, so be gentle with yourself and ease into the process.

Relationship to Balance

Notice what sustains your relationships.

Where in your life do you feel balanced?
Where do you feel out of balance?
Are you the giver or the receiver in most of your relationships?

Being in balance means something different for each of us, but overall, it means feeling grounded, clearheaded, and motivated. The heart chakra represents balance between the head and heart, self and others, giving and receiving, and being and doing. If we overextend in any relationship, we can easily feel depleted and resentful. If we don't extend enough, the relationship may not grow or flourish.

Notice if the following areas in your life feel balanced: health, relationships, work, family, friends, fun, adventure, and spirituality. Where would you like to make changes in order to restore balance?

Relationship to Gratitude

Take a moment to think about the things you are grateful for in your life. Notice how this feels in your heart chakra.

How often do you practice gratitude?
What kind or thoughtful thing did someone do for you recently?
What abilities do you have that you are grateful for?

Gratitude is thankful appreciation for what we have and what we receive, and an acknowledgment of the good in our lives. Gratitude helps us feel more connected to others and often to something greater than ourselves. This connection to people and/or to a higher power can cultivate love, generosity, and a more open heart.

In positive psychology research, gratitude is strongly and consistently associated with greater happiness. It helps people feel more positive emotions, relish good experiences, improve their health, deal with adversity, and build strong relationships.

Three Ways to Cultivate Gratitude in Your Life

- Make it a practice to tell a spouse, partner, or friend something you appreciate about them every day.
- Every day, think about something you have done well or that you appreciate about yourself.
- Keep a daily journal of three new things for which you are thankful.

Relationship to Grief

Grief is a natural reaction to loss and change. Bring your awareness to your heart chakra and notice any feelings of grief.

How often do you experience grief?
How do you process your grief?
How does grief affect your health?

Grief is a deep emotional response triggered by rejection and/or loss, such as the death of a loved one, the loss of a job, the end of a relationship, or the onset of a disease. Our individual experience with grief can vary greatly. A helpful framework for understanding grief and identifying the different emotions that can arise is the five stages of grief that Elisabeth Kübler-Ross describes in her book *On Death and Dying*.

As a Swiss-American psychiatrist and a pioneer in near-death studies, the five stages are based on Kübler-Ross's research of working with terminally ill individuals. She described the five stages as denial, anger, bargaining, depression, and acceptance.[9] She realized that these five stages were applicable to anyone experiencing a loss in their life, and the model

---

9. Elisabeth Kübler-Ross and David Kessler, *On Grief & Grieving: Finding Meaning of Grief Through the Five Stages of Loss* (New York: Scriber, 2005), 7–24.

became widely known and used. In recent years, the model has expanded to include more stages than the original five.

The stages may be a helpful tool in managing grief but may not work for everyone. We experience grief in both universal and unique ways, and no one model works for everyone. Notice if you are grieving now or recall a time in the past when you were grieving. Did you notice that you were experiencing any of these stages? Does labeling and describing the stages and the associated emotions help foster more understanding and acceptance? Remember that not everyone experiences all these stages and that the stages don't occur in a linear fashion. You may jump from one stage to another, get stuck in one for a prolonged period, or repeat the cycle many times.

Stages of Grief

Denial: "This can't be happening." Feeling numb and in a state of disbelief.

Guilt: "I should have said and done more." Feeling overwhelmed by your own emotions and needs.

Anger: "Why did this happen? Who is to blame?"

Depression: "I'm too sad to do anything." Period of isolation and loneliness.

Bargaining: Asking a higher power to intervene and give you relief in exchange for something you're willing to do.

Acceptance: "I acknowledge that this has happened and have come to understand what it means in my life now."

Return to a Meaningful Life: Feelings of hope and of possibility for the future return.

Ways to Take Care of Yourself

Allow yourself to grieve: Often we push the grief away by distracting ourselves with activities or tasks. Avoiding grief only leads to prolonging it because the emotions need to be felt and acknowledged. Give yourself the time and space to experience the emotions even when it's painful to do so.

Express your feelings: You can write about your loss in a journal or write a note to the person you've lost. You can make a scrapbook or photo album celebrating the person's life and recalling your favorite memories with them. It can be helpful to see a therapist and talk about your grief and any triggers that might be coming up from unresolved issues from the past.

Practice healthy habits: Your mind and body are connected, and physical health helps with the emotional healing process. Take walks, spend time in nature, take group exercise classes with friends. Make sure you are getting enough sleep and eating nutritious foods that provide both energy and comfort. It can be helpful to gently shift your attention from the loss and focus on self-care. Ask yourself, "What do I need to feel nourished and supported in this moment?"

Accept where you are: You are allowed to grieve for as long and as deeply as you need to, and no one can tell you when to move on. Notice if you are judging yourself and how you should be behaving rather than giving yourself the time and space to be with whatever is arising in you. Notice judgments from others and then see if you can let them go. Be loving and compassionate with yourself when you feel angry, guilty, and fearful. Let it be okay to cry or not cry, and let it be okay when you have moments of joy and laughter. Be with it all as the emotions and feelings come up. If you start to feel stuck and unable to cope with the emotions, look for a therapist to support you in this difficult time.

Relationship to Forgiveness

Take a moment and notice the role forgiveness plays in your life.

How easy is it for you to forgive?

How have you been able to forgive yourself for mistakes made in the past?

Who do you find most difficult to forgive in your life?

Forgiveness is the ability to extend understanding toward those who have wronged you. It often involves letting go of resentment, bitterness, and vengeance. It's important to remember that forgiveness does not mean forgetting the wrongdoing, denying your own pain, or excusing the transgression. Forgiveness requires us to acknowledge what happened, to name it and feel it, and then to invite some understanding and compassion toward the person or situation. The goal is to let go of your own preoccupation with the hurt, to disentangle yourself from the pain, and to find closure.

Often the process of forgiveness involves moving through the stages of grief. At first, we are in denial that it happened, then angry at the person or situation, then bargaining with them or ourselves to admit the wrongdoing or make amends, and then feeling sad and depressed. Finally, we move toward acceptance by seeing the situation for what it is and moving on.

It helps to remember that acceptance and letting go benefit you on many levels. Recognize the cost of not forgiving to your health and well-being. When you forgive, you experience fewer negative emotions, you regain your emotional stability, your heart chakra continues to grow and expand, and you experience more goodwill toward yourself and others.

Steps toward Forgiveness

Choose to forgive and stay focused on the benefits to your heart chakra.

Consider the perspective of the person you are trying to forgive. As difficult as this might be, it's an important step toward understanding and compassion.

Take responsibility for your experience and your reactions to the situation.

Consciously let go of any hostility or vengeance toward the person. You don't have to like them or condone what they did, but it's important to release toxic thoughts and feelings from your psyche. With each exhale, release the negative thought, and with each inhale, invite more love, joy, and peace into your heart chakra.

Create a plan to move forward. What are the steps you need to take to feel empowered and move on? Write a letter that you may or may not send, set clear boundaries, distance yourself from the person, or end the relationship.

Return your focus to the benefits of forgiveness and all the ways your heart chakra is growing and expanding.

Relationship to Friendships

Notice the roles friendships play in your life.

How has this dynamic changed in the last five or ten years?
How often do you make time for your friends?
What qualities do you most treasure in a friend?
In what ways are you a good friend to others?

Friendship is a mutual relationship based on honesty, trust, respect, fun, laughter, and time spent together. Friendships helps us experience love and connection in order to grow and become better people. Research shows that good relationships keep us healthier and happier. People who are more socially connected to family, friends, and community are physically healthier and live longer than people who are less connected. It's not the number of friends you have, but the quality of your connections and friendships. The best friendships have kindness and trust as the foundation and inspire feelings of warmth toward one another.

If you are feeling lonely and isolated, know that you are not alone, and don't take it personally. A new study found that almost half of Americans feel alone, and younger generations feel the most isolated. All of us get into ruts where we work too hard and don't give our existing friendships enough time and energy, or we resist cultivating new friendships.

Here are some tips from Ellen Hendriksen's book *How to Be Yourself* to make friends even if you are shy, introverted, or socially anxious.

The biggest indicator that you'll become friends with someone is physical proximity, as we tend to make friends with people we see on a regular basis. Think about the people you see on a regular basis at work, in your neighborhood, at the playground with your children, at the gym, or in your local yoga studio. Focus on the people who are friendly toward you with eye contact or a smile. Be courageous, step outside of your comfort zone, say hello, and ask a few questions. It takes about six to seven interactions with the same person to make a meaningful connection.

Once a connection is made, notice if you are opening up and sharing thoughts and feelings with this person. Disclosure helps build trust and intimacy and brings you closer. It's scary to share who you are with others, but taking little risks in opening up can lead to more fulfilling relationships. And people appreciate kind words and gestures, so when you are warm, friendly, and curious in your interactions with others, you will attract more people to you.[10]

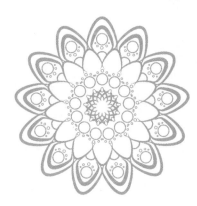

10. Ellen Hendriksen, *How to Be Yourself: Quiet Your Inner Critic and Rise Above Social Anxiety* (New York: St. Martin's Griffin, 2018), 233–253.

Relationship to Service

In the heart chakra, we move from a place of "me" to a place of "we." We continue to meet our own survival and ego needs, but we also create space for helping others. We understand the collective consciousness and take responsibility for making the world a better place for all. Our sense of compassion and empathy is awakened, and we use our energy and power to make a difference.

Ways to Serve

Regularly donate to your favorite charity.

Pray for the causes you believe in and ask for support and guidance from a higher power.

Volunteer regularly for a cause you value and for which you want to make a difference.

After a few months of serving and giving, notice the energy at your heart chakra and any changes in your relationships and life.

Questions

1. What do you love?
2. How much time do you give to what you love?
3. Do you feel love for yourself and for others in your life?
4. What opens your heart and fills you with love?
5. Are you able to forgive those who hurt you?
6. In your significant relationships, is there a balance of giving and receiving?
7. How often are you relating to others as your authentic self?

_____

_____

_____

_____

_____

_____

_____

_____

_____

_____

_____

_____

_____

_____

_____

_____

Heart Chakra Short Practice

Dog Breath to Boost Your Immune System

Sit in easy pose with your chin in and your chest out. Stick your tongue all the way out and keep it out as you rapidly breathe in and out through your mouth. The navel point moves as you pant. Continue for three to five minutes.

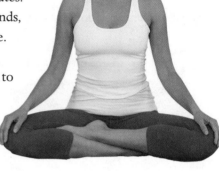

> *To end:* Inhale, hold your breath for fifteen seconds, press the tongue hard against the upper palate. Exhale. Repeat two more times.

> *Benefits:* Brings energy to your immune system to fight infection. A very healing exercise.

Spinal Flex in Rock Pose

Sit on the heels with the hands on the thighs. Inhale and extend the spine forward, exhale and push it back. Keep the shoulders over the hips and the chin parallel to the floor.

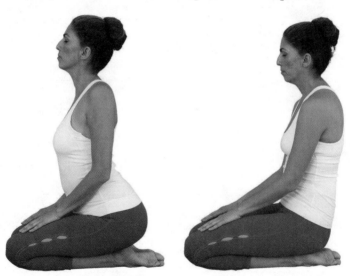

Benefits: Increases the flexibility in your upper spine.

Heart Opener

Bring the arms straight out with the palms facing forward and make tight fists. Inhale deeply and hold the breath. Pull the arms toward the heart chakra. Imagine that you are pulling a heavy weight toward you. When the fists touch the heart chakra, exhale powerfully. Repeat for a total of three to five times.

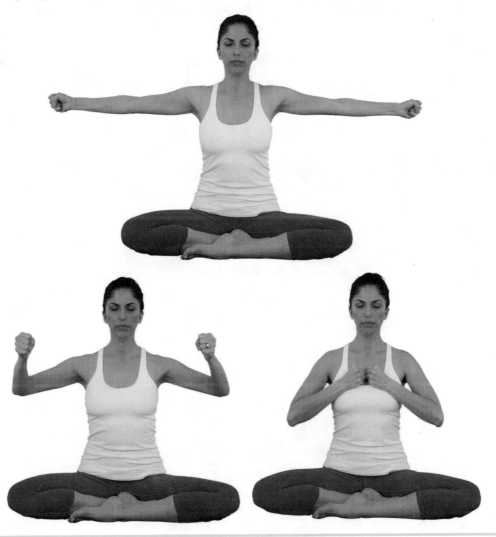

Meditation to Calm the Heart Chakra

Sit in easy pose. Bring the hands in front of the heart chakra and let the fingertips of both hands touch. Keep the wrists apart and leave space between the palms. Inhale through the nose for five seconds, hold the breath for five seconds, and exhale for five seconds. Continue for three to five minutes.

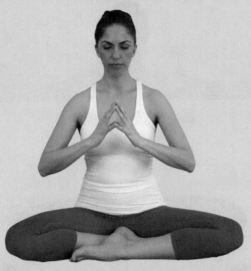

Benefits: Releases unsettling issues from the past and expands your capacity to manage stressful relationships.

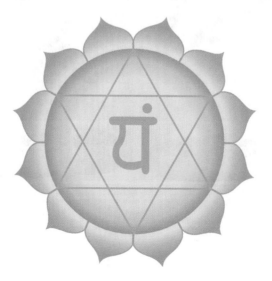

Heart Chakra Warm-Ups

Practice each pose for one to two minutes.

1. Stretch with Strap

Hold the ends of the strap and bring the arms over the head. Inhale as you bring the strap behind you toward the ground. Exhale and sweep the arms over your head and in front of your body.

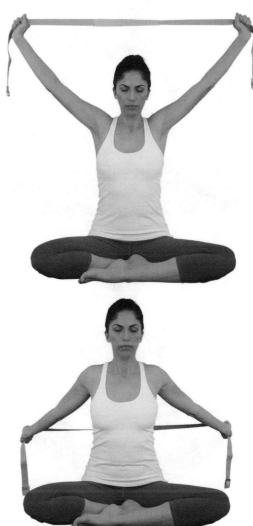

2. Arm Stretch

Wrap the right arm behind you with the back of the hand resting on the waist. The left palm grasps the right palm to feel a stretch in the arms and shoulders and across the heart. Switch sides after one minute. Breathe long and deep.

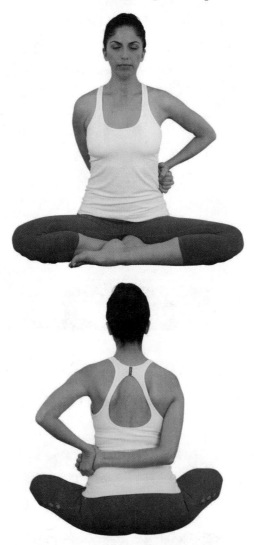

3. Spinal Flex with Arms

Stretch the arms out to the sides and inhale. Exhale, wrap the arms around you, and push the spine back with hands on shoulders. Inhale and extend the spine forward as the arms go back.

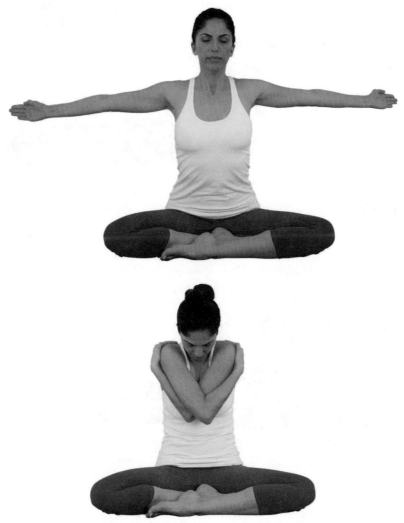

4. Spinal Twist

Place the fingers in front of the shoulders and the thumbs toward the back. Keep the elbows lifted up at shoulder height. Inhale and twist to the left. Exhale and twist to the right. Torso, shoulders, and head move together.

5. Puppy Pose

Come onto all fours and bring the forehead to the floor as you extend the arms forward. Walk your hands forward a few inches and move the buttocks halfway up and away from the heels. Drop your forehead to the floor. Press the hands down and stretch through the arms while pulling your hips back toward your heels.

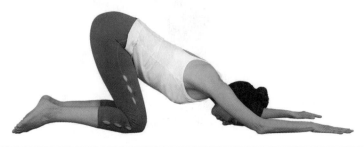

6. Thread the Needle

Come into table pose. Inhale and lift your right arm out to the side and then up toward the ceiling. Exhale and bring the right arm through the space under your left arm. Bring your right shoulder, upper arm, and side of the face closer to the floor. After one minute, switch sides.

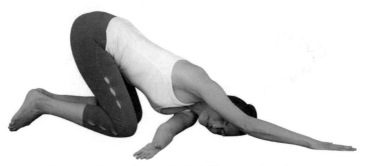

Benefits: Loosens the muscles in the back, shoulders, and neck and massages the abdominal organs.

7. Shoulder Rolls

Place the hands on the knees. Lift the shoulders up to the ears and roll them down and back for a minute. Inhale the shoulders up and exhale back down. Keep the face relaxed. After one minute, switch and inhale the shoulders up and exhale as you roll them forward and down.

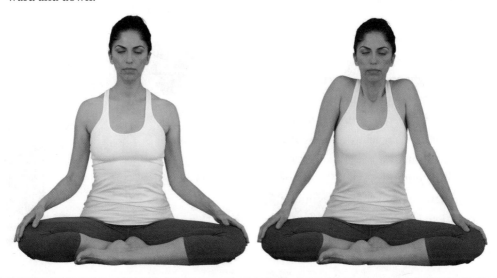

8. Bowing with Arms Interlaced in Easy Pose

Sit in easy pose. Bring your arms behind you and interlace the fingers. Inhale and stretch the arms away from you. Exhale and bring the forehead to the floor and extend the arms up toward the ceiling. Inhale and bring yourself back to sitting. Exhale back down to bowing. If the forehead does not reach the floor, you can use a bolster or blanket to support the head.

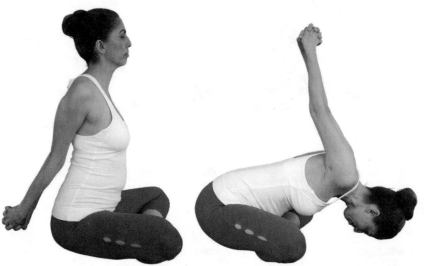

9. Camel Pose

Kneel with legs hip-width apart. Engage the abdominal muscles and move the hips forward as if you were pressing into an imaginary wall so that your thighs are perpendicular with the floor. Inhale and lift your chest upward. Exhale and slowly bend backward, sliding your hands down the back of your legs until you reach your heels. Breathe deeply. Continue to push the front of the legs and hips forward.

To come out, release the hands one at a time and gently push yourself up. Relax for one minute.

Variation: Instead of reaching for the heels, keep the hands on your lower back.

Kriya to Open the Heart Chakra

This kriya opens the heart, increases compassion, and helps drop emotional defensiveness. Its calming effect allows you to eliminate unnecessary thoughts and feelings so you can be more present and neutral.

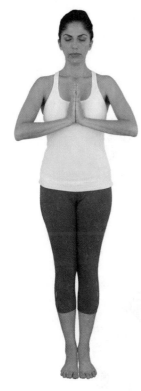

1. Stand with palms together in prayer pose at the center of the chest and do a steady breath of fire. Practice for three minutes.

To end: Inhale and hold briefly at the end.

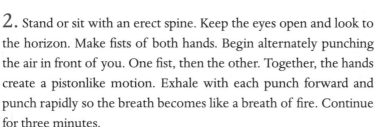
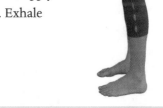

2. Stand or sit with an erect spine. Keep the eyes open and look to the horizon. Make fists of both hands. Begin alternately punching the air in front of you. One fist, then the other. Together, the hands create a pistonlike motion. Exhale with each punch forward and punch rapidly so the breath becomes like a breath of fire. Continue for three minutes.

To end: Inhale, draw both elbows back, tighten the fists, apply root lock, and suspend the breath for five seconds. Exhale and relax.

3. Stand straight, extend the arms out to the sides, and begin to make big circles with both arms at the same time. Inhale as they come forward and up, and exhale as they go back and down. Continue for two minutes.

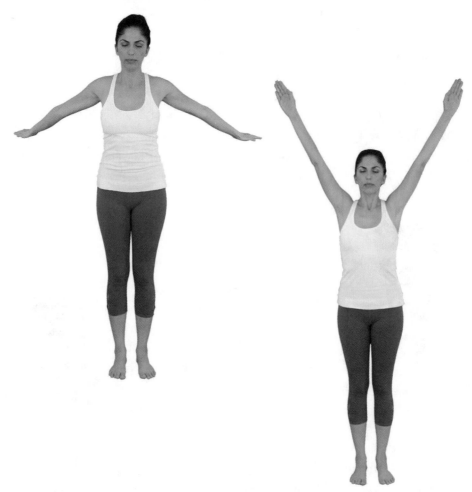

To end: Inhale and stretch both arms straight up over the head. Exhale and relax.

4. Sit straight. Interlace the fingers with the thumb tips touching. Position the hands four to six inches in front of the chest with both palms facing down. Lift the elbows to the same level. Inhale as you lift the hands up to the level of the throat. Exhale as you sweep them down to the level of the navel. Create a steady pumping motion with a powerful breath. Continue for three minutes.

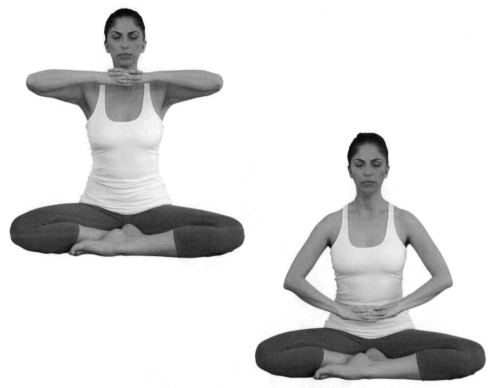

To end: Inhale, bring the hands to the level of the heart, and suspend the breath for ten seconds. Exhale and relax.

5. Stand or sit with a straight spine. Place the hands beside the shoulders with elbows by your sides and palms facing forward. Close your eyelids halfway and fix your gaze downward. Begin to slowly inhale and exhale. Your breath should be equal on the inhale and the exhale. Mentally repeat the following primal sound scale on both the inhale and exhale:

Saa Taa Naa Maa

Universe, Creation, Death / Dissolution, Rebirth (represents the cycle of life)

Press the thumb tips to each fingertip sequentially as you chant:

Saa: thumb to pointer finger;

Taa: thumb to middle finger;

Naa: thumb to ring finger;

Maa: thumb to pinkie finger.

Continue for three to five minutes.

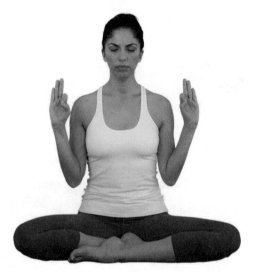

To end: Inhale and exhale.

6. Sit with a straight spine. Block the right nostril gently with the index finger of the right hand. Inhale slowly through your left nostril, exhale slowly through rounded lips. Match the duration of the inhale and exhale, with each one lasting about ten seconds. Continue with this slow breathing pattern for three minutes. Then relax and follow the natural flow of your breath for another two minutes.

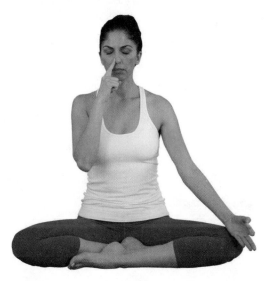

Relax for seven to ten minutes. Rest on your back with the legs straight and the feet splayed out to the sides. Make sure you are warm and comfortable as you begin this relaxation. Soften the ankles, calves, and shins. Let the thighs melt into the floor. Allow your breath to find its own natural rhythm while softening the navel area. Let the spine sink into the earth. Relax the chest, shoulders, arms, and hands. Visualize a beautiful, spiraling, green light around your heart center. Invite new levels of love, compassion, and acceptance. Soften the muscles in the neck and throat. Let your entire face soften. Visualize rays of green light showering your entire body with unconditional love and healing.

Meditation for Gratitude

In this meditation, you simply sit and allow all the blessings of your life to fall into your cupped hands. Feel yourself merging with the light of those blessings. This meditation will help you awaken to and express your gratitude for the kindness and love of the people in your life.

Posture

Sit comfortably in easy pose with a straight spine and a gentle neck lock.

Mudra

Cup your hands together at the heart chakra and rest the upper arms against your ribs.

Eye Focus

Eyes are closed.

Visualization

Visualize all the blessings in your life. Meditate on the divine flow of love in your heart and in your life.

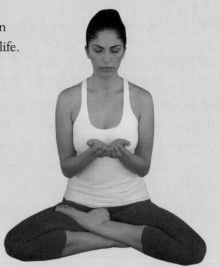

Breath

Breathe deeply and feel yourself merging with the light of all of those blessings.

Time

Continue for three to ten minutes.

To End

Inhale deeply and relax.

Meditation to Awaken Love and Compassion

This meditation opens the heart chakra to deeper feelings of love, compassion, and acceptance. This mantra is chanted to create inner peace so you can project outer peace.

Posture

Sit in easy pose.

Mudra

Place the left hand at the heart chakra, palm facing four to six inches away. Keep the fingers stiff but not tight. The forearm is parallel to the ground. The right arm is straight, resting on the knee. Hold the right hand in active gyan mudra, with the forefinger curled under the thumb and the other fingers straight but joined.

As you concentrate on the hand, you may feel a warm energy moving through the hand to the heart chakra.

Breath

Natural breathing.

Eye Focus

Focus at the tip of the nose.

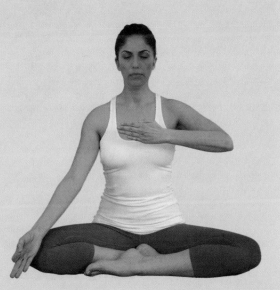

Mantra

Sat Narayan Wahe Guru (True sustainer, Indescribable wisdom)
Hari Narayan Sat Nam (Creative sustenance, True identity)

Time

Practice for three to ten minutes.

To End

Inhale, hold briefly, and exhale. Meditate with open awareness as your heart chakra adjusts your feelings with the boundaries of the self.

Music Recommendation

Ajeet Kaur, *Sacred Waters*

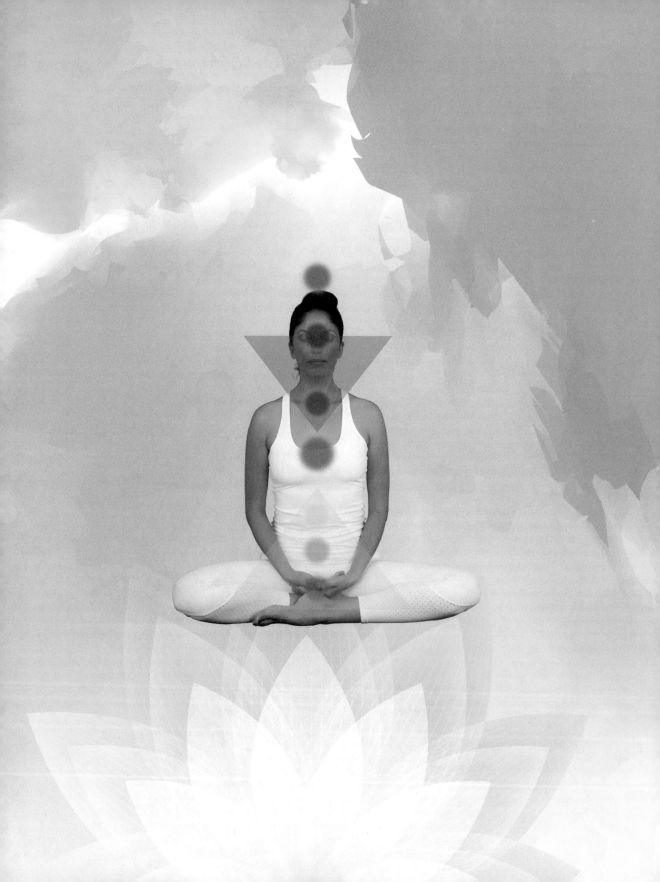

Part 4
The Higher Chakras

The higher chakras, also called the higher triangle, include the fifth, sixth, and seventh chakras. These three chakras have more subtle and esoteric qualities and connect us with higher consciousness and awareness.

The fifth chakra is the center of communication, creative expression, deep listening, and relationship with truth. When the fifth chakra is balanced, we feel in rhythm with life, comfortable sharing our feelings and thoughts, tuned in to our inner voice, able to silence our inner critic, and able to use our words to elevate and uplift others.

The sixth chakra is our connection with intuition, guidance, strategic thinking, and clear vision. The sixth chakra is also our primary means of cultivating a relationship with our soul. Soul is that part of us that is neutral, focused on learning and growing, able to transcend the many dualities in life, and balances the head and heart. A balanced sixth chakra sees the many possibilities in life and is guided by the light of the soul rather than the mental calculations of the ego.

The seventh chakra is the center for thinking, awareness, spirituality, and nonattachment. When the seventh chakra is balanced, we become aware of our thoughts without reacting to them. We cultivate spiritual practices to experience peace, learn to let go and become less attached, and trust in the process of life.

The higher chakras connect us with the spiritual realms and our place in the world in relation to the big picture. Why are we here? What are we meant to do? What are the guiding principles of our lives? The gifts of the higher triangle are meant to bring us closer to our divine nature. The higher triangle is more open to receiving ideas from the spiritual realms and manifesting those ideas on the earth plane. The mantra of the higher triangle is that we are spiritual beings having a human experience.

The lower triangle, the heart chakra, and the higher triangle are equally important to our well-being. Each chakra can help us connect more deeply with our true nature. We value the chakras closest to the earth as much as the chakras closest to the heavens. The goal is to honor our life on Earth and all that it entails, and honor our spiritual nature and the energy of the infinite.

Let your words uplift and elevate.

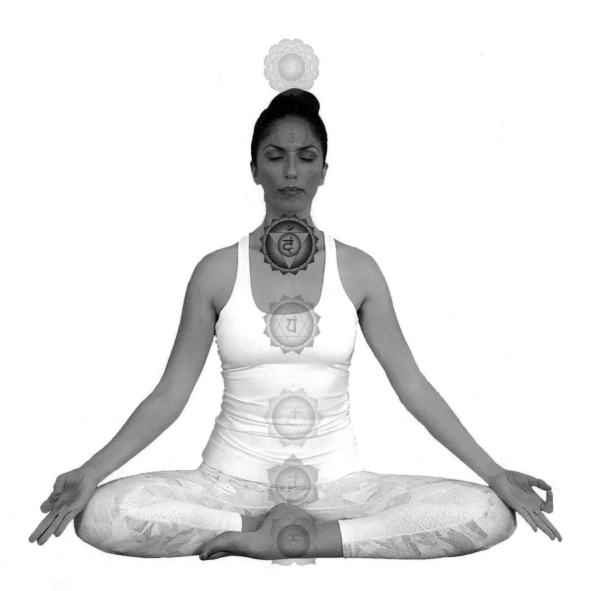

Chapter 6

THROAT CHAKRA (5th Chakra)

Sanskrit Name:	Visuddha (Purification)
Main Issues:	Communication, creativity, truthfulness, and lies
Element:	Ether
Location:	Throat, neck, jaw, mouth, teeth, and ears
Color:	Blue
Goals:	Effectively communicate, express your highest truth, and live creatively

Balanced Energy

- Clear and effective communication
- Mindful listening
- Creative and expressive
- Truthful and kind
- Connected to your highest truths
- Tuned in to the cycles and rhythms of life

Deficient Energy

- Tension in the neck and jaw
- Fear of speaking
- Speaking with a small or weak voice
- Excessive shyness
- Tone-deaf and poor rhythm

Excessive Energy

- Excessive talking and interrupting
- Inability to listen or be silent
- Gossiping
- Dominating voice
- Excessively critical of self or others

Healing Practices

Chanting

Singing

Journaling

Cranial-sacral therapy

Expressive theater and dance

Commit to truthful communication

Silence

Affirmations

I trust my inner voice.

I share my feelings with
ease and comfort.

I live my truth.

I am creative and expressive.

My words have power and impact.

I listen to understand.

The Symbol

The symbol of the fifth chakra is a circle with sixteen petals that represent the sixteen vowels of the Sanskrit language. In the middle is a downward-pointing triangle signifying a channel to our higher consciousness and soul. Within the triangle is a circle that represents the moon and suggests a purified mind.

Some versions of the symbol include a white elephant called Airavata. The elephant is depicted with seven trunks, which are said to represent the seven chakras. The seed mantra is **Ham.**

Relationship to Ether

Take a moment and notice what makes you feel vast and expansive.

What is your relationship with the ether element?
How do you experience subtle energy?

Ether is the limitless space or cosmic void in which everything exists. Ether is associated with spirituality, openness, freedom, communication, and expansiveness. It tends to be still, light, and ever-present. Looking up at the sky connects you with the openness and vastness of the ether element. Being mindful of the space between your inhale and exhale and the space between your thoughts connects you with the ether element.

Ether is part of the subtle energy system that connects your mind to infinity, stillness, and peace. Ether connects you to the universal consciousness.

Relationship to Communication

Think about how you communicate your inner truth with the world.

Are you more comfortable speaking or listening?

Do you know why you prefer one over the other?

Do you feel heard when you speak?

What are you wanting from others when you communicate—to be acknowledged, heard, understood, loved?

Are you aware of the impact your words have on others?

The throat chakra gives you the gift of communication and the ability to use your unique voice to express your creative essence and your truth. The throat chakra is the vehicle through which you speak, share feelings and thoughts, listen to others, and listen to your own inner voice. When the throat chakra is open and flowing, you feel relaxed in the areas around your shoulders, neck, and jaw. You are comfortable listening to others and sharing your feelings and thoughts. When you speak, your words have purpose and meaning, and you are not talking just to talk.

When the throat chakra is balanced, you listen deeply, take in what the other person is saying, and notice nonverbal cues. You are able to stay in the moment and focus on what the person is sharing with you.

Communication is a skill that improves with practice. In order to bring healing to the throat chakra, become aware of your communication style. Notice if you talk incessantly, if you hold back from talking, if your words are intense and critical, or if you agree with others just to avoid conflict. Start by bringing awareness to your conversations and notice what you notice. The simple act of noticing without judging can create change and healing.

The throat chakra is a powerful tool in creating meaningful relationships with others. When you share what is inside of you with others, it can create intimacy and trust in the relationship. If you keep all your ideas and feelings to yourself, it creates congestion, anxiety, confusion, overwhelm, and isolation. Look for ways to express what's longing to be shared, and notice if you feel more peace and harmony in your energy system. Try journaling, drawing, dancing, singing, and chanting as creative outlets to keep the mind clear and the emotions balanced.

Notice these five levels of listening so you can practice listening to truly understand.

Levels of Listening Model[11]

1. Someone is speaking to you, but you don't hear a single word.

2. You listen at the start, but you're reminded of something (more) interesting, and you miss the rest of what the person says.

3. You're attentive and engaged but waiting for a chance to ask questions and make comments.

4. You're listening to everything being said and not interrupting, but you're thinking about how it relates to you.

5. You are listening with curiosity and suspending your own filters of judgment, values, and needs, and trying to appreciate what it means in their world.

Tips for Conscious Communication

- *Nonverbal Communication:* The majority of what you say and what you hear is communicated through nonverbal cues. Be aware of your posture, breath, body language, and intention when you are communicating. Your presence speaks louder than your words. Stay connected to your navel chakra when you communicate and stay grounded in your body.

- *Allow for Pauses and Silences:* Pauses give you time to think about what you are going to say and to fully take in what has been said. Cultivate this inner awareness to slow down and be mindful of what the other person needs and what you want to share. Notice how comfortable you are going deep into the essence of the conversation.

- *Balance Inquiry with Advocacy:* When you are listening, ask clarifying questions and be curious about what the other person is saying and sharing. Powerful questions are thought-provoking, invite reflection, and help the other person find deeper meaning and expand possibilities. If you are only advocating for your own point of view, it limits the conversation. If you only ask questions and don't share your own thoughts and feelings, it creates an imbalance in the relationship. Sharing requires courage and vulnerability and is necessary to strengthen and deepen any relationship.

---

11. R. Stephen Covey, *The 7 Habits of Highly Effective People: Powerful Lessons in Personal Change* (New York: Simon & Shuster, 1989), 252–253.

Command Your Communication with the Pinkie Finger Mudra

Press down the nail of the pinkie finger with the thumb for about a minute. Your entire sense of communication will align with your intention. The pinkie finger represents the planet Mercury, which denotes the principles of communication, thinking patterns, and reasoning. This mudra creates the capacity to clearly and intuitively communicate your message.

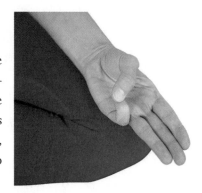

From Which Chakra Are You Communicating?

Each chakra has a different communication style and voice. Notice if you can converse in all the styles listed below or if you favor a specific style. Is your use of language always loving or always direct? Do you take a moment to notice the intention behind your communication and which chakra is fueling it?

Chakra Eight: Expansive

Chakra Seven: Divine

Chakra Six: Intuitive

Chakra Five: **Direct**

Chakra Four: Loving

Chakra Three: **Powerful**

Chakra Two: **Seductive**

Chakra One: **Primal and Instinctual**

Relationship to Truth and Lies

Notice the role truthfulness and lies play in your life.

How often do you lie and tell half-truths?

Can you tell when others are being truthful with you?

Were you forced to keep family secrets or were secrets kept from you?

How often do you actually mean what you say?

The throat chakra is the vehicle through which we express our truth or hide behind lies. Truth is defined as words and actions that are aligned with your most authentic self.

Lies come in many forms. You can tell yourself lies and live in ways that do not resonate with your true nature. You can keep secrets, overlook truths, and fail to speak up at crucial times. All these actions put you out of sync with your life force energy and your core truths. Truth has a resonance that allows all parts of your psyche to be in harmony. The work of the throat chakra is to express your truth in your words and actions and stay committed to your truth in the face of challenges.

If you deceive yourself and others with lies, the throat chakra becomes drained or stagnant. Lying takes energy, and a pattern of lying depletes the throat chakra and leads to fatigue. Lying, gossiping, and hurtful words all weaken the throat chakra and negatively impact the thyroid and parathyroid glands. The thyroid gland is located in the front part of the lower neck and produces hormones that impact metabolism, weight management, and the development of the nervous system. The parathyroid glands are small glands in the neck located behind the thyroid gland and regulate calcium levels in the blood. Kundalini Yoga sets and meditations for the throat chakra can help balance the energy in this chakra and bring healing to the thyroid and parathyroid glands.

Trust that you have the courage and strength to be kind and honest in your conversations. People can handle your truth, and you can handle theirs. Communicating at this deep and authentic level takes practice.

Practicing Sat Kriya for three to five minutes every day can build courage and help you communicate more effectively and authentically.

During Sat Kriya, you chant the mantra *Sat Nam* (I am truth and truth is my essence). This mantra connects you with your pure life force energy and gives you the strength and conviction to be true to yourself.

Relationship to Creative Expression

Creativity is a form of self-expression and a basic urge to make an offering to the world. Notice the role creative expression plays in your life.

How do you express your creativity in your daily life?

What forms of creative expression call to you? (Writing, dancing, drawing, singing, acting, etc.)

What stops you from expressing yourself and sharing your creativity with others?

Creative expression is accessible to you in your everyday life. You don't have to be a painter, dancer, or performer to experience it. You can be creative in your daily life with how you dress, decorate your house, cook, garden, host a party, and so much more.

The throat chakra is the vehicle that allows you to express your feelings, desires, passions, and ideas. Listen to the creative ideas and inspirations you've been ignoring and let them come out to play. Trust that these ideas are coming to you for a reason and that you are meant to share them with the world. Let your desire to make the world a better and brighter place be greater than any fears or doubts. If an idea comes to you, grab it with all your energy, commit to it, and share it with the world.

Relationship to Your Inner Critic

Imagine befriending your inner critic, observing the negative comments, and then redirecting your thoughts to a more supportive outlook.

Are you aware of your inner critic voice?

How often do you believe this inner critic?

What helps you distinguish the voice of your inner critic from the voice of your supportive self?

The inner critic is a voice in your head that lets you know when you've made a mistake and gone off course. Ideally, the inner critic helps you get back on track, but too often it's way too harsh and condemning.

The voice of your inner critic is composed of all the internalized critical judgments you've heard in your life from parents, teachers, and peers. It's a running commentary on everything that is wrong with you and your decisions. The inner critic can erode your confidence and wear down your willpower. We can't get rid of the inner critic, but we can learn to tame it and neutralize it with the nurturing voice within. Just as we have an inner critic, we also have an inner nurturer that uplifts us and connects us with our inner strengths.

Pay attention and recognize the voice or voices of your inner critic, listen to the messages, and create space between you and this voice. Your inner critic is not always truthful or accurate. It has a distorted view of reality based on the past. Learn to question and challenge the inner critic voice. It can help to name your inner critic and give it a personality. This helps you recognize the voice more quickly and then dismiss the criticism.

The critic's voice is a habitual pattern created in the mind and can be replaced by new patterns that are affirming and empowering. Know that the inner critic shows up when are you are creating change in your life, taking risks, and moving toward growth and empowerment. During these times of change, growth, and transition, recall memories of times when you successfully overcame a challenge and/or achieved your goal. Turn the volume up on the voice of the inner nurturer, remember the voices of your supporters, and create space in your mind for these affirming, positive voices.

One more technique to use to tame the inner critic is to create a folder that you fill with significant experiences or achievements. It can be an actual folder or an online folder. My folder has pictures of all my travels and big hiking trips. When my inner critic shows up and refuses to leave, I turn to this folder and look through the images, and within a few minutes, my perspective shifts, and the inner critic loses its grip on my psyche. The folder reminds me of my strength and resiliency and makes me feel that I can face any challenge.

When the inner critic shows up, pause and listen to the message. Then ask yourself, "Whose voice is this? Is this true? How do I know it's true? What else could be going on?" And then, "If it is true, then what's the worst-case scenario? [Be specific.] How can I use my inner strengths to deal with this scenario? What are the resources I can bring in?"

Relationship to Mantra

Notice your relationship to sound, music, and chanting.

How do you feel about your voice?
How often do you sing and chant?
What sounds relax and elevate you?

Mantras are sounds that help the practitioner become absorbed in deep states of meditation and transformation. Mantras are known to have the power to awaken and balance the chakras. Mantras are sound vibrations created by the ancient yogis to focus the mind, awaken consciousness, transcend the ego, and connect with the divine. This is accomplished by the repetition of a mantra, either aloud or in silence. The mantras in this book are from the Kundalini Yoga tradition and are in the language of Gurmukhi.

When you chant a mantra, eighty-four meridian points located on the hard and soft palate of the mouth are stimulated. These meridian points send messages to the hypothalamus, which is connected by blood vessels to the pituitary gland. The pituitary gland, known as the master gland, regulates hunger, thirst, body temperature, and sleep. The pituitary gland also triggers the regulation of mood, emotional behavior, and sexuality. The special patterns of the mantras stimulate the hypothalamus to change the chemistry of the brain, which results in many positive states of mind.

Chanting mantras creates a relationship with your voice. Accepting and loving your voice creates deep healing for the throat chakra. Take every opportunity to chant, sing, and project your voice out into the world. When you chant, you create an inner vibration that fosters peace and harmony.

The chakras are associated with specific mantras called seed sounds or bij mantras. Chanting these sounds brings balance to each chakra. Chant each sound rhythmically for a minute while visualizing that particular chakra. You can go in order and chant each mantra for one minute or just focus on one for a few minutes.

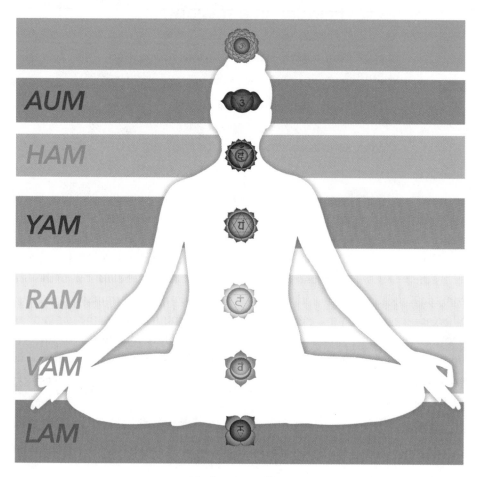

Chakra 7: **Silence**

Chakra 6: *AUM*

Chakra 5: *HAM*

Chakra 4: *YAM*

Chakra 3: *RAM*

Chakra 2: *VAM*

Chakra 1: *LAM*

My Top Mantras to Create Inner Harmony

When I feel out of sync with my environment and my mind feels scattered, I hit the pause button and chant one of these mantras to reset.

Sa Ta Na Ma

"Life, death, rebirth, infinity,"

by Nirinjan Kaur;

to increase intuition, balance the brain hemispheres,
and connect you to the cycles of life.

Kal Akaal

"Undying,"

by Sirgun Kaur;

removes negativity.

Humee Hum Brahm Hum

"We are we. We are God,"

by Gurusangat Singh;

to open the heart chakra and connect you with spirit.

Dharti Hai Akash Hai

"Earth and Ether,"

by Meditative Mind;

calls on your highest spirit.

Bhand Jameeai

"Meditations for Transformation,"

by Gurunam Singh;

honoring the divine feminine.

Communication Cleanse and Reboot

Communication is key to sustaining healthy and happy relationships. Devote one day a week to these practices so that your communication is mindful, impactful, and compassionate:

• Abstain from lying, gossiping, complaining, and criticizing. When you catch yourself doing any of these, take a deep breath, let it go, and begin again. Let go of judgment.

• Practice your nonpreferred mode of communication. If you are usually the talker, listen more. If you usually listen, talk and share more with others.

• Listen to understand, be curious, and be interested.

• When communicating your feelings, use "I" statements and be kind with your words.

• Chant the mantra *Sat Nam, Sat Nam, Sat Nam, Sat Nam, Sat Nam, Sat Nam, Wahe Guru* for ten minutes, and then sit in silence for five minutes and notice what you notice.

• Notice the feedback you receive from others when you use these practices.

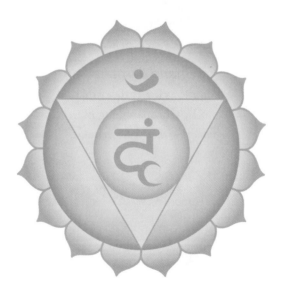

Questions

1. What were the communication patterns in your family? Were you encouraged to share your feelings and thoughts? Did you feel heard?

2. What are you longing to hear?

3. What are you longing to express to the world?

4. How clear and honest are you in your communication with yourself and others?

5. How often are you critical of yourself and others?

6. Where and when do you feel most creative and expressive in your life?

_____

_____

_____

_____

_____

_____

_____

_____

_____

_____

_____

_____

_____

_____

Throat Chakra Short Practice

Dog Breath

Sit in easy pose with your chin in and your chest out. Stick your tongue all the way out and keep it out as you rapidly breathe in and out through your mouth. The navel point moves as you pant. Continue for three to five minutes.

> *Benefits:* This breath helps clear the body and the throat chakra of toxins. It helps oxygenate the blood. It will help clear the energy at the throat chakra.

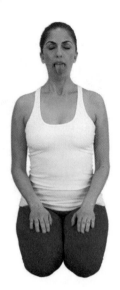

Cat Cow

Come onto all fours with your wrists directly under your shoulders and your knees directly under your hips. Make sure there is space between the knees. Inhale and drop the spine down and lift the head up. Exhale and round the spine upward and drop the head down. Continue at your own pace for one to two minutes.

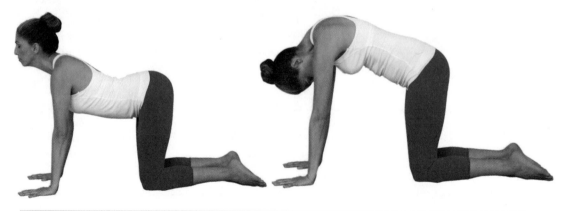

Neck Turns with No and Yes

Sit in easy pose and turn your head to the left and to the right. As you move your head, feel a connection to your heart chakra. Begin to chant the word *no* as you move your head side to side. Practice saying no out loud to the things that drain your energy. Play around with different tones as you chant no. Practice for one minute.

Then move your head up and down and chant yes. Practice saying yes to the things that light you up and open your heart chakra. Play around with different rhythms and tones as you chant yes. Continue for one minute.

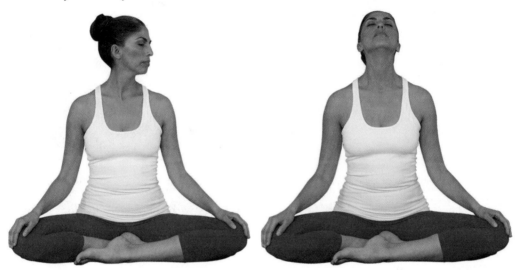

Benefits: Opens and clears the throat chakra, connects you to your voice, and makes you aware of things to avoid or to embrace.

Chanting

Pick a mantra and chant it for three to five minutes. As you chant, listen to your voice with love and compassion, and connect with the vibration of the mantra. Here are some of my favorites for the throat chakra.

Wha Hay Guru, "balances the ether element"—Nirinjan Kaur, *Prem Siri*

Har Haray Haree, "guidance and prosperity"—Kamari & Manvir, *Aquarian Technology*

Ang Sung Wahe Guru, "connects you with the divine"—Gurudass Kaur, *Longing to Belong*

Throat Chakra Warm-Ups

Practice each pose for one to two minutes.

1. Spinal Flex

Sit in easy pose. Grab your
knees and extend your spine
forward and back. Keep the
shoulders over the hips. Inhale
as you extend forward and
exhale as you press back.

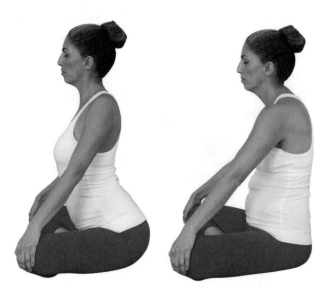

2. Spinal Twist

Sit in easy pose and place the hands on the shoulders with the fingers in front of the
shoulders and the thumbs in the back. Inhale and move your waist, shoulders, and neck
to the left in one smooth motion. Then exhale and move to the right. Continue side to
side with a powerful breath.

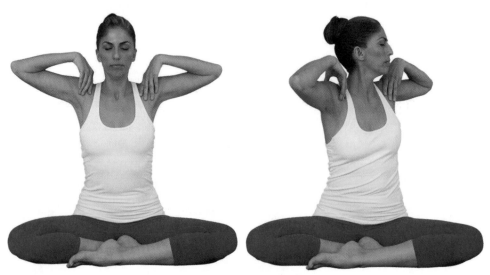

3. Elbows Up

Sit in easy pose and rest the hands on the shoulders. Inhale and lift the elbows up toward the ceiling. Then, exhale and lower the elbows to shoulder height. Continue alternating between the two movements. Lift from the rib cage as you inhale the elbows up.

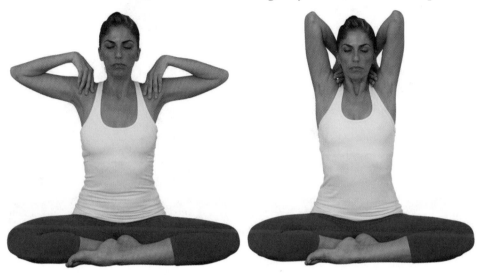

4. Shoulder Shrugs

Sit in easy pose and place the hands on your knees. Lift both shoulders up and roll them back with long, deep breaths for one minutes. Then lift both shoulders up and roll them forward for one minute.

5. *Figure 8 Neck Rolls*

Draw a figure 8 with the nose in one direction for one minute. Move slowly with long, deep breaths. Then, reverse the direction.

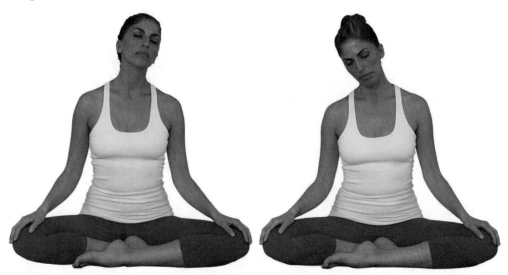

6. *Cat Cow*

Come onto all fours and place the wrists under the shoulders and the knees under the hips. Make sure there is space between the knees. Inhale and drop the spine down and lift the head up. Exhale and round the spine upward and drop the head down. Continue at your own pace.

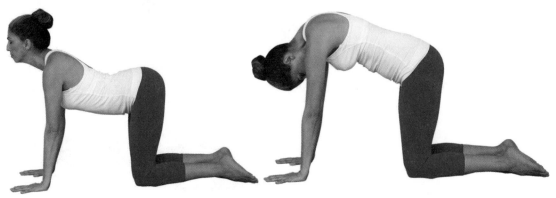

7. Cow Pose to Triangle Pose

Come onto all fours with your wrists directly under your shoulders and your knees directly under your hips. Inhale and drop the spine down and lift the head up. Exhale and push into the hands and feet and straighten the legs into triangle pose. Inhale back down into cow pose and then exhale into triangle pose. Continue alternating between the two poses.

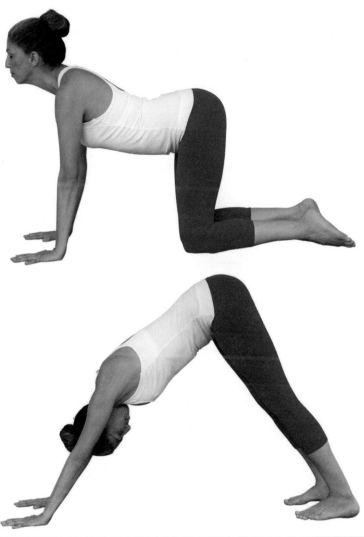

Kriya to Balance the Throat Chakra

This kriya is a complete workout for the thyroid and parathyroid glands. It also helps the thymus gland and the immune system. Over time, this practice will help you express your truth and enhance your communication so that your words are clear and uplifting for others.

1. Stand with feet together or hip-distance apart, and bring the hands to prayer pose. Inhale and extend the arms straight out 60 degrees, tilt the head back, and look at the ceiling. Exhale and bring the head back to neutral and the hands back to prayer pose. Create a steady motion with the breath. Continue for two to three minutes.

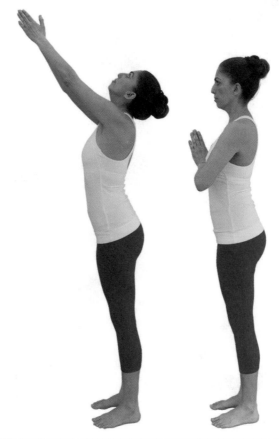

2. Sit in rock pose and extend both arms out to the sides, parallel to the ground, with palms facing up. Turn your head to the left while breathing in deeply. Turn your head to the right while breathing out. Mentally breathe in Sat and breathe out Nam. Continue for two to three minutes.

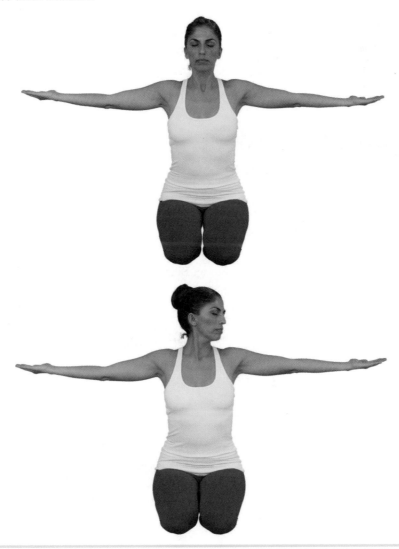

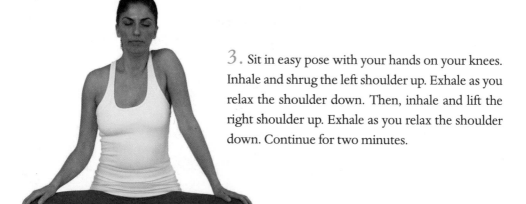

3. Sit in easy pose with your hands on your knees. Inhale and shrug the left shoulder up. Exhale as you relax the shoulder down. Then, inhale and lift the right shoulder up. Exhale as you relax the shoulder down. Continue for two minutes.

4. Sit in rock pose and stretch both arms forward parallel to the ground with the palms facing down. Lift the head up and back to a comfortable angle and look up at the ceiling. Begin breath of fire. Continue for two to three minutes. Then inhale, bring the neck back to neutral, and exhale.

5. Sit in easy pose and interlace your hands in venus lock at the base of the lower back. Bring your head and chin down toward the sternum. Begin breath of fire. Continue for two to three minutes.

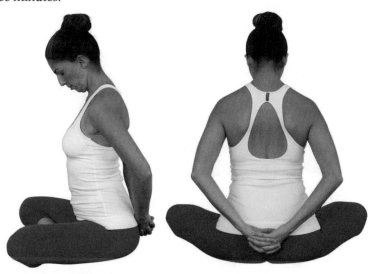

6. Sit in easy pose, lengthen the spine, and lift the chest up slightly. Rest the hands on the knees in gyan mudra. Breathe in completely, turning your head to the right. Breathe out totally, turning it to the left. Mentally vibrate Sat Nam. Continue for one to two minutes.

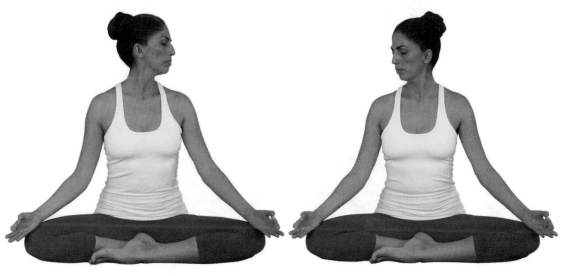

7. Sit with your legs stretched straight out and gently press the feet forward. Place the hands on the ground behind you and lean back 30 degrees. Gently lift the head up and back and look toward the sky. Start a steady, long, deep breath. Continue for two to three minutes. Then inhale and straighten the neck. Relax.

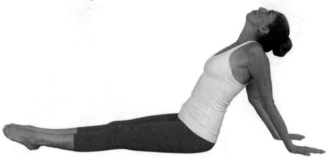

8. Sit in rock pose and stretch the arms overhead to hug the ears. Interlace the fingers, cross the thumbs, and stretch the index fingers up. Keep the elbows straight. Inhale as you lean forward 30 degrees. Exhale as you lean back 30 degrees from center. Continue this motion for one to three minutes.

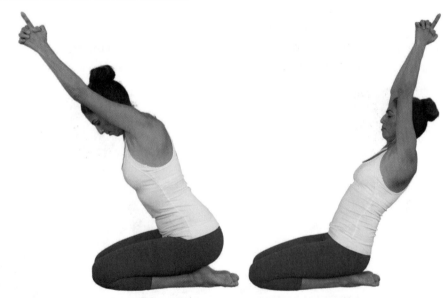

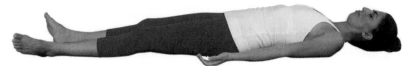

Relax for seven to ten minutes. Relax on your back and feel the support of the earth. Soften all the muscles in your legs. Relax the hips and buttocks. Let go of any effort. Let your breath flow freely. Soften the chest, shoulders, arms, and hands. Relax all the muscles in your throat and neck. Visualize a beautiful blue light around your neck, mouth, jaw, and ears. Imagine the throat chakra as a clear channel of energy expressing your truth and creativity. Imagine floating in the clouds, in perfect balance with the vastness of the cosmos.

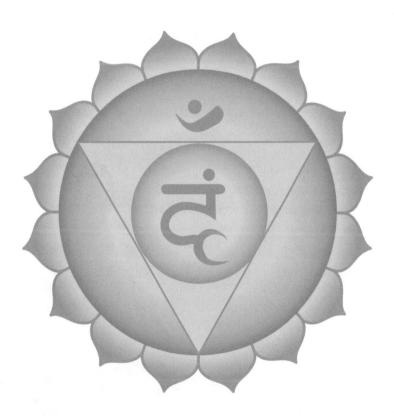

Meditation for Effective Communication

This meditation develops communication between the chakras. It combines the energies of the lower and the higher chakras to create integration. A regular practice of this meditation expands your capacity for effective communication so that your words have mastery and impact.

Posture

Sit in an easy pose with a light neck lock.

Mudra

Make buddhi mudra with both hands (by touching the thumb tips to the tips of the little fingers). The other fingers are relaxed but straight.

Eye Focus

The eyes are closed.

Mantra

Sa Re Sa Sa, Sa Re Sa Sa, Sa Re Sa Sa, Sa Rung,
Har Re Har Har, Har Re Har Har, Har Re Har Har, Har Rung
Sa is the infinite, the totality, and the element of ether.
Har is the creativity of the earth and the power of manifestation. These sounds are woven together to create complete totality.

Time

Practice for ten to thirty minutes.

To End

Inhale, exhale, and relax.

Music Recommendation

Nirinjan Kaur, *Mantras for Prosperity*

Meditation for Clarity and Creativity

Practice this meditation to experience more clarity and prosperity as it balances the negative and positive minds, creating a neutral state so that you can effectively visualize the things that will support your life and spiritual growth. It is said that this meditation and breath pattern will connect you with the source of creativity that is in your heart, solve the problem of how to make a lucrative living, and satisfy your soul.

Posture

Sit in easy pose.

Mudra

Raise the arms in front of the body with the forearms parallel to the ground at shoulder-height. Bend the elbows so the fingers can point toward each other in front of the throat center, palms facing down. Bend the ring and pinkie fingers under the thumbs on the palms. Extend and touch the tips of the index and middle fingers to the tips of the opposite hand.

This mudra stimulates the energies of Saturn and Jupiter, which represent the polar approaches to learning—through mistakes and discipline, and through expansion and exploration. Both Saturn and Jupiter are called upon to act through the fifth chakra for creativity and command.

Breath

Inhale through the nose for two to three seconds. Hold the breath in for five seconds. Then exhale completely through the nose for ten to fifteen seconds.

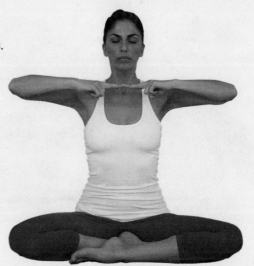

Eye Focus

Keep the eyes slightly open.

Time

Practice for ten to thirty minutes.

To End

Inhale deeply, exhale, and relax.

Awaken your intuition.

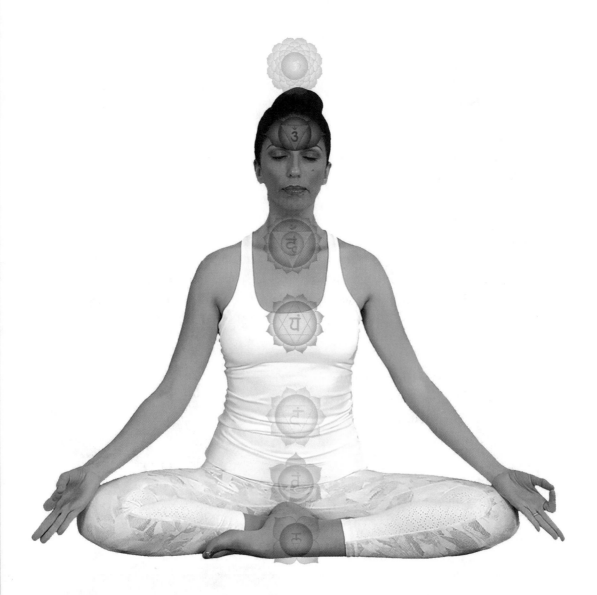

Chapter 7
THIRD EYE CHAKRA
(6th Chakra)

Sanskrit Name:	Ajna (Command Center)
Main Issues:	Intuition, soul, and illusion
Element:	Light
Location:	Brow point, eyes, pituitary gland
Color:	Indigo
Goals:	To see clearly, to connect with your intuition, and to discover your life purpose

Balanced Energy

- Intuitive
- Insightful
- Reflective
- Imaginative
- Focused
- Good memory
- Remembers dreams

Deficient Energy

- Unimaginative
- Difficulty visualizing
- Insensitive
- Excessive skepticism
- Denial of reality
- Inability to see all possibilities
- Inability to remember dreams

Excessive Energy

- Difficulty focusing
- Excessive fantasizing
- Intrusive memories
- Hallucinating
- Obsessing
- Having nightmares
- Delusional thoughts

Healing Practices

Look for the good in each person and see the divine in everyone

Create more harmony and beauty in your physical surroundings

Give your eyes a feast by going to an art museum or spend time in nature

Pay attention to your dreams and start a dream journal

Read and watch inspirational books and movies

Create a vision board

Affirmations

I open myself to my inner guidance and wisdom.

I trust that my highest good is unfolding.

I am intuitive and aligned with the light of my soul.

I seek wisdom and guidance in all situations.

I see clearly and am open to all possibilities.

The Symbol

The symbol for the Ajna chakra is a circle encompassing the mantra Om, which represents spiritual unity.

There are only two petals at the sixth chakra; they represent the duality in life. Duality symbolizes the opposing forces in life, such as masculine and feminine, the sun and moon, happy and sad, and heaven and Earth. The petals often bear the letters *Ha* and *Ksa*. These petals connect the right and left lobes of the pituitary gland and are linked to the right and left hemispheres of the brain. The ida and pingala nadis meet at the sixth chakra, and this merging can help us transcend duality and experience oneness with all things in life.

At the center of this chakra is an inverted triangle, representing reality, consciousness, and joy. Above the triangle is a shining crescent moon, signifying the pure white color that is often seen when the third eye opens to the radiant light within. The seed mantra is **Aum.**

Relationship to Beauty

The sixth chakra is energized and awakened by all things beautiful.

What brings your eyes pleasure?

What makes your eyes feel energized and inspired?

How do you allow yourself to see the beauty within you?

Time spent looking at beauty in nature, in art museums, and at the wonder and magic of your own imagination awakens and replenishes the sixth chakra. When you look at something beautiful, you experience a sense of awe. Awe takes you beyond yourself and connects you with something greater than your limited perspective. Looking at majestic mountains, a starlit sky, or the vast ocean awakens and energizes your sixth chakra and merges your energy with the energy of the cosmos.

Relationship to Your Soul and Intuition

> The sixth chakra transcends duality and connects you with the light of your soul and the voice of your intuition.
>
> *How often do you reflect on your life experiences?*
>
> *Do you recognize the patterns in your life and the lessons learned?*
>
> *What is your relationship to your intuition?*
>
> *How do you connect with the light within you?*

The soul is the part of you that serves the highest good, looks beyond the ego needs of self-protection and self-promotion, and connects you with your life purpose. In the sixth chakra, you focus on the entirety of the self and recognize your own divine nature and the divine nature of others. Once you recognize that your true nature is both human and divine, you experience the light of your consciousness and see more clearly. You recognize the duality within yourself and in life, but you are no longer swayed by that duality. You understand the difference between being and doing. Your self-worth no longer comes from accomplishment and achievement, but rather from the attitude, perspective, and outlook of what is inside of you. You shift your focus from outward appearances to experiencing inner peace, joy, harmony, and love.

The mantra *Wha Hay Guru* means moving from darkness to light and connecting with the indescribable wisdom of your soul. The repetition of this mantra clears the mind of darkness and ignorance and connects you with your light and radiance. Darkness and ignorance represent our judgments, filters, and assumptions that everything we see, think, and feel is real. The mantra *Wha Hay Guru* encourages you to shine a light into the darkness and see the deeper meaning in all your life experiences.

Intuition connects you with the gift of clairvoyance, which translates to clear seeing. It is said that intuition comes from wisdom, and wisdom comes from life experiences. Intuition is the ability to go beyond the analysis of the intellectual mind and use the resources of your senses, your heart, and your soul. Your soul wants you to see your life as a spiritual journey. Your intuition sends you messages to direct you on your spiritual journey and learn the lessons you came here to learn. Intuitive messages challenge you to take risks, continue learning and growing, cultivate a relationship with the divine, and understand why you are here and what you are meant to be doing to serve the greatest good.

The sixth chakra directs you to turn inward and connect with the light, love, and joy within—to live from a place of inner peace and harmony and transcend the games of the ego by changing your perspective from fear to love. The ego feels pain and suffering while the soul transcends these emotional dramas. When you are connected to your soul, you are guided by your higher awareness and wisdom, and you can handle the challenges in life with grace.

The work of the sixth chakra is to let go of the attitude *I am not enough*, because this perspective only fosters fear, anxiety, cynicism, fatigue, and negativity. If this attitude is lodged into your psyche, then nothing you do will be enough. If you change your attitude to *I am light, love, and divine*, your presence and being are more than enough. The most important work of the sixth chakra is becoming aware of how you see yourself, working toward seeing yourself as pure love and light, and feeling worthy of receiving and giving the gifts of life. When you see yourself as love and light, you can see others in the same way. *My light sees the light in you and my soul connects with your soul.* This way of seeing each other elevates and uplifts relationships.

The mantra *Namaste* means "the light in me honors the light in you." *Namaste* is a beautiful yogic salutation to experience a soul connection with others.

Relationship to Confusion

Confusion arises when there is a lack of understanding and a feeling of uncertainty.

How often do you feel confused in your life?
What are the fears that arise with the confusion?
Are there certain areas in your life where there is persistent confusion?

The pituitary gland is located at the sixth chakra. Known as the master gland, the pituitary gland is responsible for the secretion of serotonin, which is an important chemical and neurotransmitter believed to regulate anxiety, happiness, mood, and sexual desire. Low levels of serotonin have been associated with depression.

During times of confusion, people fluctuate between dueling thoughts of *Yes, take the risk, you'll succeed,* or, *No, don't take the risk, you'll fail.*

It becomes a tug-of-war in your mind that, over time, is exhausting because you're not sure what to believe. Between these two opposing thoughts is the place of the meditative or neutral mind, which understands both perspectives and moves forward with a level of detachment regarding the outcome. The perspective shifts from *What am I going to gain or lose in this situation?* to *What am I going to learn? How will this align me with the light of my soul?*

Kundalini Yoga offers many yoga sets and meditations that stimulate the pituitary gland so that you can rise above confusion, gain clarity, and trust more in the process of life.

Meditation to Free You from Confusion and Depression

Sit in easy pose with the arms straight out to the sides at shoulder height with the palms down. Start to flap the hands from the wrists. Breathe long and deep. Continue for three minutes.

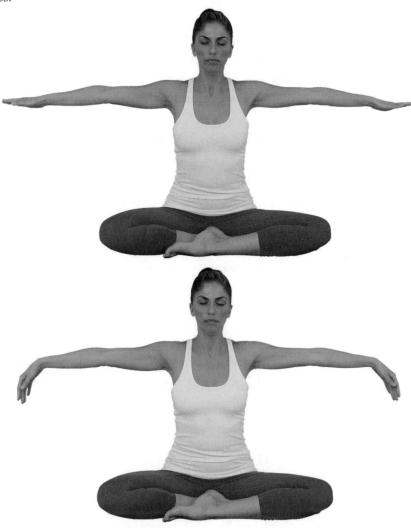

Benefits: Lifts confusion and depression.

Relationship to Dreams

Dreams bring you images from your unconscious mind and are an important part of the sixth chakra.

How often do you remember your dreams?
What are your dreams trying to communicate to you?

Dreams communicate with images and symbols. Paying attention to your dreams can reveal significant insights into your life. Start a dream journal and notice any recurring images, people, and conversations. Notice what your unconscious is ready to share with you and how these dreams can help you see yourself and your life more clearly.

Relationship to Illusion

Notice your relationship with your eyes and how clearly you see yourself and the world.

How do you see yourself?
How do you want others to see you?
Does your inner reality sync up with your outer image?
What are you refusing to see in your life?

Ajna means to perceive and to command. To perceive is to see or recognize a pattern. In this context, to command means to hold a picture in your mind as a guiding model for manifestation.

From a young age, you are inundated with images telling you how to look, think, and behave. It's easy to fall into a pattern of following the guidelines outlined by your family and culture. If you believe the guidelines and norms prescribed by them, you tend to be more at peace.

If you are at odds with the prescribed norms, you experience inner turmoil and conflict. You may repress your true identity in order to be accepted and loved. Which people and what situations trigger you to hide your true nature? What are the fears that arise?

Healing the sixth chakra requires clearly seeing who you are on a deep level and sharing this self with others.

Illusion fixates your mind on what "should be" and obscures your reality. Notice how often you hear messages in your mind about how you should look, what you should be doing, who you should be with, and the type of work you should be doing. All the "shoulds" in your life obstruct your energy and your happiness. Instead, open your eyes to the beauty that is in you and your life. Notice if you recognize the "should" voice as your own or someone else's. Is it the voice of your inner critic or a critical parent? Give yourself permission to be yourself and connect more deeply with what you love and value instead of what you think you should love and value. Also check in with trusted friends when you feel stuck in your illusions. Share your observation with them and be open to their feedback.

Relationship to Your Life Purpose

Imagine sitting on a mountaintop and looking down at your life from this vantage point and notice if any revelations come to you about the purpose and meaning of your life.

What are your gifts?
What do you most love doing?
What inspires you?

Your life purpose is a unifying theme that draws on your unique gifts and talents and combines them with activities that bring you joy and fulfillment while serving others. Your life purpose can help guide decisions and create meaning and value in your life.

To discover your life purpose, you have to go beyond your ego needs of self-promotion and self-preservation and connect with the journey of your soul. Your ego tends to turn away from your purpose because it might be dangerous to your reputation or cause you to look ridiculous in the eyes of others. In fact, a big life purpose threatens the part of you that wants to stay small and safe.

Life purpose is something that has always been part of you, and it's a quality that comes naturally and easily to you. Your life purpose is not always clear but can be ascertained when you pay attention to the moments in life when you feel the most fulfilled. These significant life experiences are clues to what you truly care about and who/how you want to serve. Ultimately, your life purpose will help you honor what you love to do and move you away from what drains you.

Recall memories from your childhood, teenage years, early adulthood, and recent experiences. Notice when you felt alive, full of spark, happy, satisfied, and most excited. Take a moment and write down some memories from these age periods:

Conception to 11 years old

Adolescence: 11 to 21 years old

Young Adult: 21 to 40 years old

Maturity: 40 to 66 years old

Elder: 66 years and older

Taking Time to Reflect

1. What activities were common among the memories in your lifetime?

   _____

   _____

   _____

   _____

2. What was it about the particular experience that made you so happy?

   _____

   _____

   _____

   _____

3. How were you serving others in these situations?

   _____

   _____

   _____

   _____

4. What are the specific gifts / qualities you were born with and that come naturally to you in your life?

_____

_____

_____

_____

Create Your Life Purpose Statement

A life purpose statement is short, simple, and inspiring. Examples include the following:

- Teach from my heart.
- Create safe and healing spaces for others to learn and grow.
- Love and be loved.
- Help others connect with the light within.
- Inspire the artist within all of us.

My life purpose is …

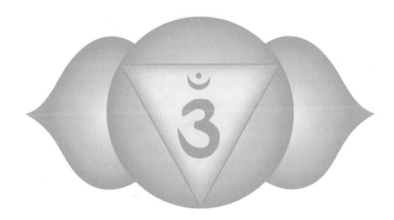

Beautiful, Bountiful, and Blissful

The sixth chakra helps you float above the specifics of any situation and see the expansive possibilities. This beautiful mantra lifts you above the limitations of time and space and connects you with your expansive nature. This mantra invites you to see yourself and others as beautiful, bountiful, and blissful.

Chant this mantra when you want to uplift your mind and connect with the light of your soul.

I am the light of my soul
I am beautiful, I am bountiful, I am bliss
I am I am

Music Recommendations:

Sirgun Kaur and Sat Darshan Singh, *The Music Within*

Ajeet Karu, *Darshan*

Questions

1. What helps you connect with your intuition?

2. When was the last time you took a leap of faith?

3. What is your relationship with your soul?

4. Is there something you don't want to see that is going on in your life?

5. How can you look at the challenging experiences in your life and distill wisdom from them?

6. Do you recognize what is valuable and beautiful within you?

7. How are you able to visualize the future and envision all the possibilities?

_____

_____

_____

_____

_____

_____

Third Eye Chakra Short Practice

Palming Eye Exercise

Rub your hands together for ten to fifteen seconds until they feel warm and then gently place your hands over your eyes, with the fingertips resting on the forehead. The palms aren't touching the eyes directly but simply covering the area around the eyes to create darkness. Close your eyes, breathe deeply, relax, and enjoy this break from visual stimulation. Continue as long as it feels soothing. When done, gently remove the hands from the face and slowly open the eyes.

Bowing

Sit on the heels with the knees wide apart. Inhale and come up onto the knees and stretch the arms up to 60 degrees with the eyes open and looking up at the ceiling. Exhale and bring the palms and forehead to the floor. Continue for one to three minutes. Make sure the forehead touches the floor.

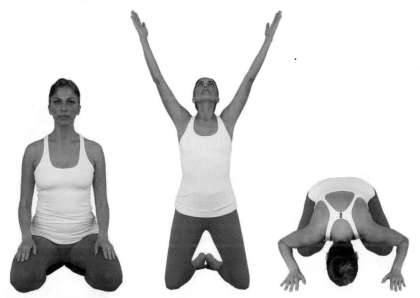

Benefits: Brings the head and heart into balance and stimulates the pituitary gland. Relaxing and elevating.

Dolphin Pose

Come onto the floor on your hands and knees. Set your knees directly below your hips and your forearms on the floor with your shoulders directly above your wrists. Interlace your fingers and firmly press your palms together as you press your forearms into the floor. Curl your toes under, then exhale and lift your knees away from the floor. At first, keep the knees slightly bent and the heels lifted away from the floor. Continue to press the forearms actively into the floor. Hold your head between the upper arms; don't let it hang or press heavily against the floor. Continue to lengthen your tailbone away from the pelvis and lift the top of your sternum away from the floor. Hold for one minute.

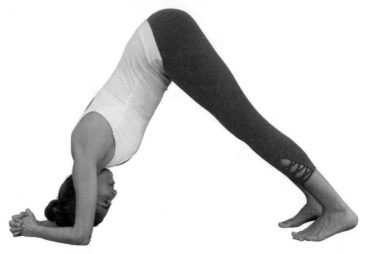

Benefits: Relief from headaches, insomnia, fatigue, and mild depression.

Meditate at the Third Eye Point

Sit in easy pose with a light neck lock. Eyes are closed and focusing upward at the middle of the brow. Bring your hands into prayer pose and rest the tips of the thumbs at the brow point. Continue for one to three minutes.

    Benefits: Stimulates the pituitary gland and enhances intuition.

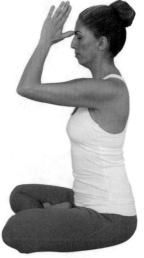

Third Eye Chakra Warm-Ups

Practice each pose for one to two minutes.

1. Mountain Pose

Stand with the feet together. Keep the shoulders down and the spine long.

Keep the head balanced over the heart and the heart balanced over the belly button. Bring the hands into prayer pose. Breathe long and deep. Connect with your foundation, your roots, and the healing, grounding energy of Mother Earth.

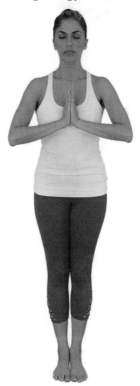

2. Arm Stretch with Strap

Hold the ends of a strap or scarf and bring the arms in front of the body. As you inhale, keep the arms straight, and stretch them over your head and behind you. On the exhale, bring the arms back to the front of the body. Hold the strap as wide as you need to.

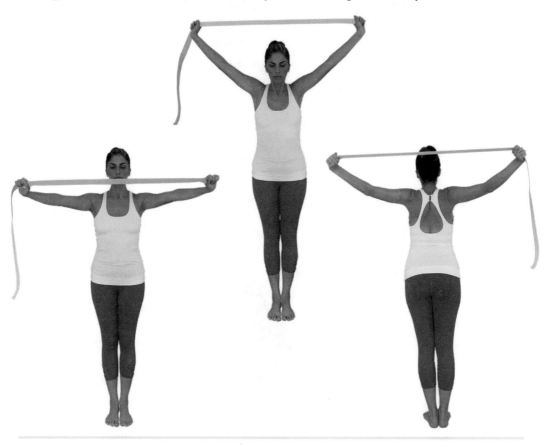

2. Arm Stretch with Strap (continued)

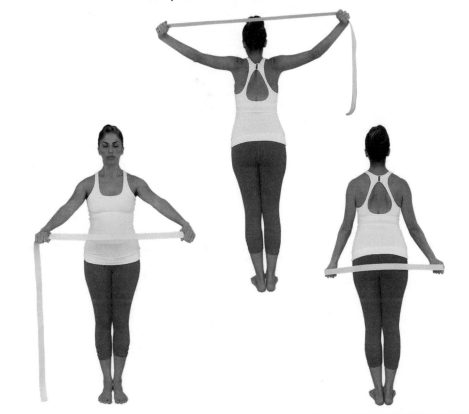

3. Forward Fold

Stand with the feet hip-distance apart. Inhale and stretch the arms up toward the ceiling with the palms flat. Exhale, hinge from the hips, and bring the fingertips to the floor.

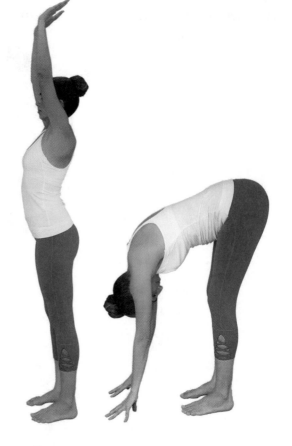

4. Triangle Pose

Begin in table pose with the wrists under the shoulders and hips over the knees. Push into the hands and feet and lift the body into a triangle. Lengthen the spine, draw the shoulder blades toward each other, relax the head, push the legs away from you, and press the heels toward the earth. Breathe long and deep.

5. Cat Cow

Come onto all fours and place the wrists under the shoulders and the knees under the hips. Make sure there is space between the knees. Inhale and drop the spine down and lift the head up. Exhale and round the spine upward and drop the head down. Continue at your own pace.

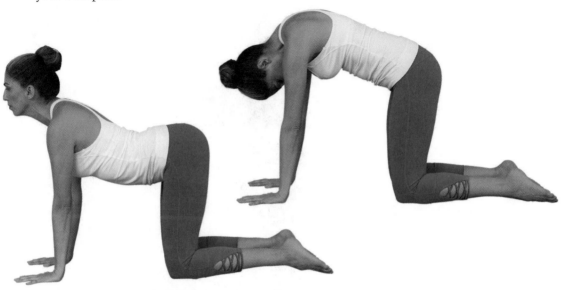

6. Puppy Pose

Sit on the heels, bring the forehead to the floor, and extend the arms forward. Walk your hands forward a few inches and move the buttocks halfway up and away from the heels. Drop your forehead to the floor. Press the hands down and stretch through the arms while pulling your hips back toward your heels.

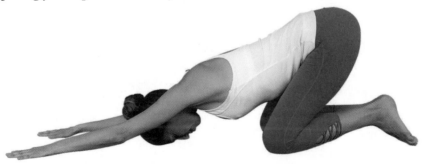

7. Child's Pose

Come into child's pose with arms stretched out in front and the palms together. Forehead rests on the floor. Place the forehead on the ground and stretch the arms overhead, keeping the palms together. Meditate at the brow point and connect with your inner light.

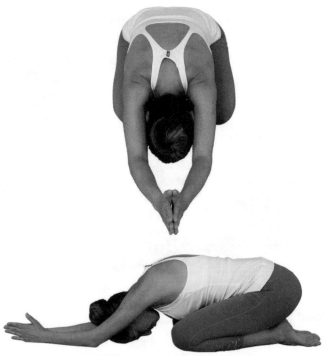

Kriya for the Third Eye Chakra

The sixth chakra is associated with the third eye, which gives you clarity, wisdom, focus, and depth. The three major energy channels—ida, pingala, and the sushmuna—meet at the third eye and help the mind transcend duality to see clearly. This kriya stimulates the pituitary gland and connects you with your intuition, which is your ability to listen deeply, see clearly, and follow the bliss of your soul.

1. Bowing. Sit on the heels and bring the hands behind you and interlace the fingers. Inhale and bring your forehead to the floor, making sure the brow point touches the floor, and extend the arms up 90 degrees or as high as you can. Exhale and lift the head up and bring the arms down. Continue for one to three minutes.

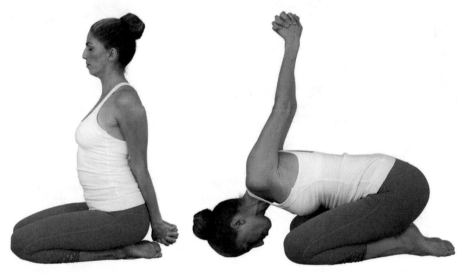

Variations: Place a block or bolster under the head. Sit in easy pose if rock pose is uncomfortable. Use a strap if shoulders are tight.

2. Cat cow. Come onto the hands and knees. Inhale and drop the spine down while the head looks forward. Exhale and push the spine up and drop the head down. Continue for one minute.

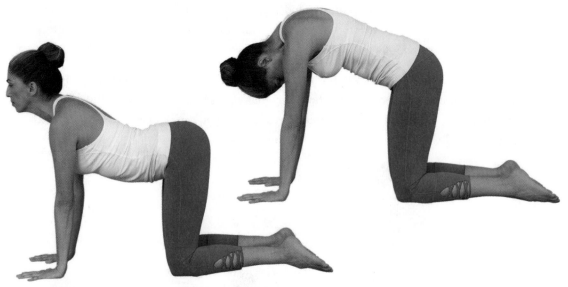

Silently chant the affirmation, *"I see clearly."*

3. Cat cow kicks. Staying on the hands and knees, inhale as you extend the left leg behind you, drop the spine down, and look forward. Exhale, engage the core, and bring the head and knee toward each other. Continue for one minute. Switch sides.

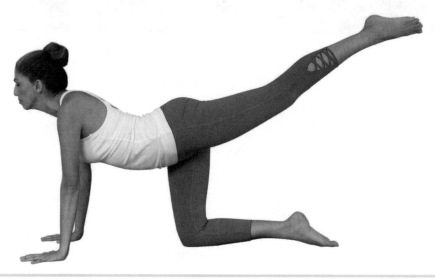

4. Lie down on your back. Bring the arms out on the floor in a *T* shape and lift the legs up to 90 degrees. Exhale, bend the knees, and let the feet come down toward the buttocks and sweep the arms up toward the ceiling with the palms four inches apart. Inhale and start again.

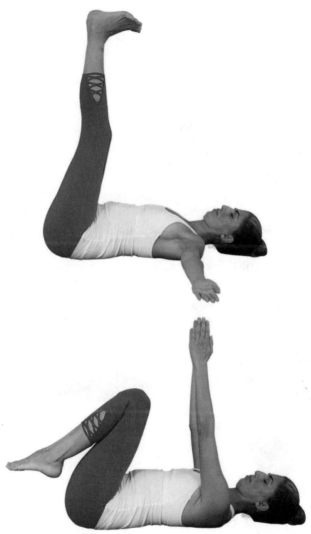

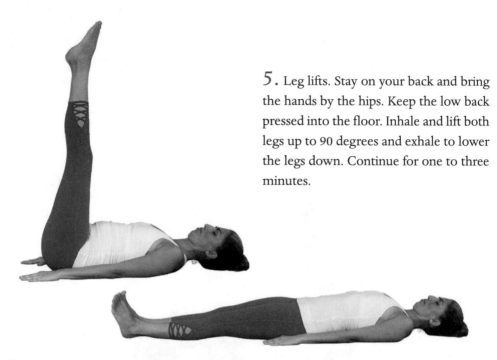

5. Leg lifts. Stay on your back and bring the hands by the hips. Keep the low back pressed into the floor. Inhale and lift both legs up to 90 degrees and exhale to lower the legs down. Continue for one to three minutes.

6. Dynamic cobra. Lying on the stomach, bring the hands under the shoulders and keep the heels together or hip distance apart. Inhale as you push up, arch the spine, and keep the hips on the ground. Exhale down. Continue for one minute. Increase the speed and continue for another minute.

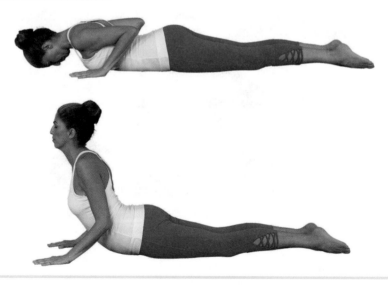

7. Arm lifts. Sit in rock pose or easy pose and bring the arms out to the sides. Inhale and lift the arms up until the palms touch. Exhale and lower the arms down. Focus on lengthening up from the spine, circulating the energy from the navel point, and building your auric field. Keep the shoulders and face relaxed. Continue for one to three minutes.

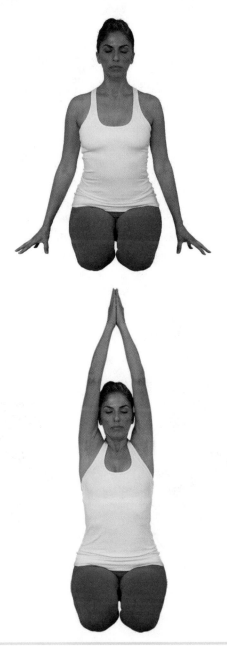

8. Kundalini lotus. Sit with the legs in front of you. Grab the ankles or the big toes and balance on your buttocks. Engage the core, keep the chest lifted, and raise the feet off the ground. Slowly start to straighten both legs. One variation is to keep the knees bent while holding on to the backs of the thighs. Breathe long and deep. Continue for one to three minutes.

9. Frogs. Squat down with the knees out to the sides and the fingertips on the floor. Head looks forward. Exhale, press into the fingertips, straighten the legs, and bring the head toward the knees. Keep the heels off the ground. Inhale and squat back down with the head looking forward. Continue for twenty to fifty repetitions.

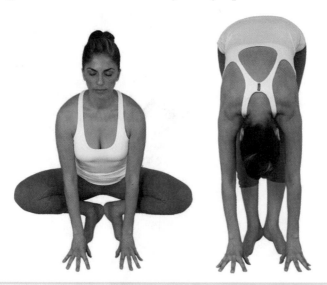

10. Bowing. Sit on the heels and bring the hands behind you and interlace the fingers. Inhale and bring your forehead to the floor (making sure the brow point touches the floor) and extend the arms up 90 degrees or as high as you can. Exhale and lift the head up and bring the arms down. Continue for one to three minutes.

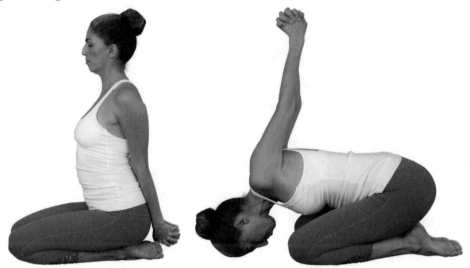

Relax for seven to ten minutes. You may want to place an eye pillow over the eyes as you ease into relaxation. Lie on your back and begin to soften your entire body. Relax the top of the head and the entire face. Allow the lips to be slightly parted and for the breath to find its natural rhythm. Let go of any effort. Soften the neck, shoulders, arms, and hands. Allow the chest and the shoulder blades to release and melt into the ground. Relax the stomach muscles, hips, legs, and feet. Imagine being showered in a beautiful indigo light that is balancing your third eye and connecting you more deeply with your intuition.

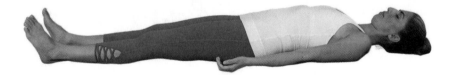

Meditation for Connecting with Your Soul

This meditation helps you consciously connect with your soul and opens your mind to experiencing peace and prosperity, while avoiding the games of the ego.

Posture

Sit on the floor in easy pose, keep the spine straight, and apply a gentle neck lock.

Mudra

Relax your upper arms by the sides of your rib cage and bring the hands up to the level of the heart. Interlace the fingers with a grip somewhat tighter than normal.

Eye Focus

The eyes are focused on the tip of the nose.

Mantra

Ardas Bhaee Amar Das Guru Amar Das Guru Ardas Bhaee Ram Das Guru Ram Das Guru Ram Das Guru Sachee Sahee

Guru Amar Das is the energy of grace and hope when there is no hope. Guru Ram Das is the energy of miracles, healings, and blessings.

Breath

Natural breathing.

Time

Ten to thirty minutes.

To End

Powerfully and deeply inhale, raise the arms over your head, and hold for ten to fifteen seconds. Exhale powerfully. Repeat two more times. Then lower your arms, sit still for one minute, and feel the vibrations of the mantra.

Music Recommendation

Nirinjan Kaur, *From Within*

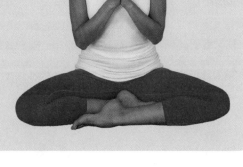

Meditation for Awareness and Inner Peace

This meditation helps open the flow of kundalini energy. The new awareness will give you the ability to overcome the challenges in your life and feel more peaceful and secure. Visualize the energy of liberation as you move the hands up toward the heavens and the energy of manifestation as you move the hands down toward the earth.

Posture

Sit in easy pose with the spine straight.

Mudra and Movement

Put the hands flat together in prayer pose at the navel point. As the mantra starts with *Sa Re Sa Sa*, bring the hands up toward the heart, about four to six inches in front of the body. As you pass the heart chakra, begin to open the hand mudra to make an open lotus by the time the hands reach the level of the brow point. The open lotus has the base of the palms together. The little fingertips touch, the thumb tips touch, and the rest of the fingers are spread open.

As the mantra begins *Har Re Har Har*, turn the fingers to point down, with the back of the hands touching. It is a reverse prayer pose. Slowly bring this mudra down the chakras in rhythm with the music until the fingertips reach the navel point on the sounds *Har Rung*. Then turn them around and begin again.

Mantra

Sa Re Sa Sa, Sa Re Sa Sa, Sa Re Sa Sa, Sa Rung
Har Re Har Har, Har Re Har Har, Har Re Har Har, Har Rung

This mantra dissolves adversity and releases any obstacles to achieving a relationship with your higher consciousness. It also takes away negativity from within so you can dwell in peace.

Breath

Let the breath regulate itself.

Time

Practice for ten to thirty minutes.

Music Recommendation

Nirinjan Kaur, *Mantras for Prosperity*

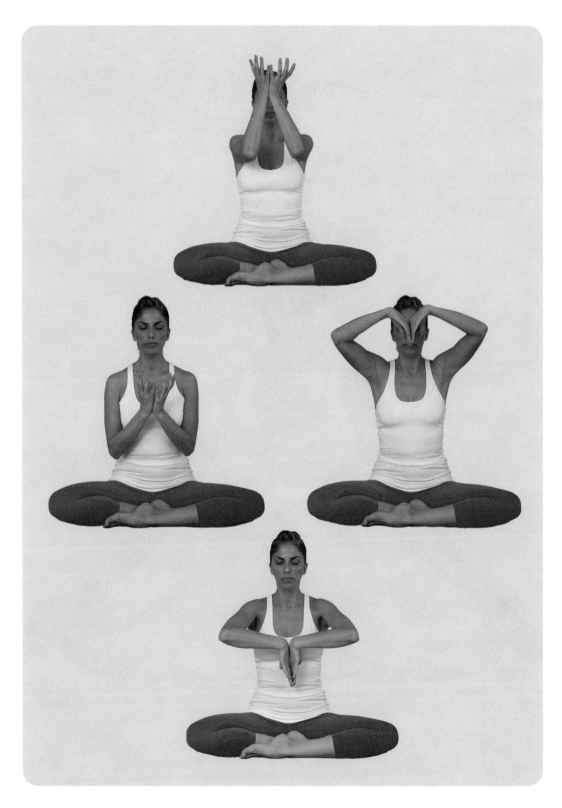

Surrender to bliss.

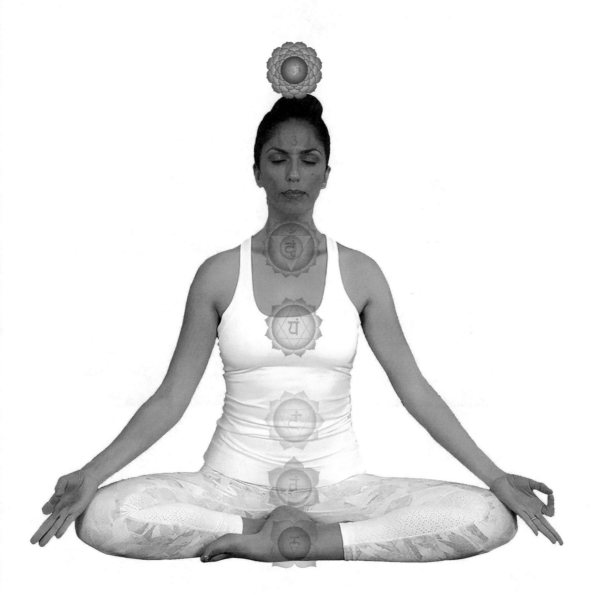

Chapter 8
CROWN CHAKRA (7th Chakra)

Sanskrit Name:	Sahasrara (Thousandfold)
Main Issues:	Awareness, analysis, beliefs, and spirituality
Element:	Thought
Location:	Top of the head and pineal gland
Color:	Purple
Goals:	Awareness, expansion, bliss, meditation, and connection with the divine

Balanced Energy
- Open-minded
- Aware
- Calm and peaceful
- Curious
- Spiritually guided
- Independent thinker

Deficient Energy
- Close-minded
- Cynical
- Rigid belief system
- Learning difficulties
- Depressed
- Bored and apathetic

Excessive Energy
- Fanatical
- Overly intellectual
- Spiritual addiction
- Dissociation from body and the world
- Inability to manifest
- Confused and frustrated

Healing Practices

Meditate

Pray

Spend time in contemplation and silence

Take a class in something intellectually or spiritually stimulating

Release limiting beliefs and explore your true beliefs about yourself and your life

Read spiritual books

Affirmations

I am open to new ideas.

The world is my teacher.

My mind serves the light of my soul.

My life is divinely guided.

I am at peace with my life.

The Symbol

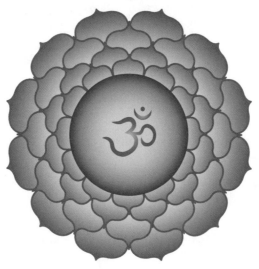

The symbol for the crown chakra is a lotus with a thousand petals, with the number one thousand representing infinity and completion. The petals are arranged in twenty rows, and each row of fifty petals contains the fifty characters of the Sanskrit alphabet. The ancient texts say the petals are turned downward and the petals are believed to be white.

The circle represents the full moon and the awakening of the mind. Some versions of this symbol also contain a circular moon and a luminous triangle that lies inside of the moon region.

Relationship to the Neutral Mind

Notice how you make decisions in your life and how content you are with the outcomes of these decisions.

What criteria do you use when making major life decisions?

How often do you fall into analysis/paralysis?

What is a life decision you are currently grappling with, and how can the three functional minds help you make this decision?

Kundalini Yoga describes the mind as having three functions: negative, positive, and neutral. Negative mind warns you of the dangers in a situation, and positive mind recognizes rewards and opportunities. Then neutral mind computes the input from the positive and negative minds and makes a decision based on nonattachment to the outcome and in service of the highest good.

Cultivating a deeper relationship with the neutral mind moves you beyond duality and into a place of wisdom. Neutral mind directs you toward growth and learning without any attachment to a specific conclusion. The positive, negative, and neutral minds are developed differently in each person. Befriend your three minds to make decisions with more confidence, ease, and peace.

Negative mind is the fastest mind and the first to react. Its job is to protect you. It asks, *What is the danger in this situation? What do I need to consider? How do I protect myself?*

Positive mind is expansive and looks for possibilities in all situations. It is constructive and takes risks. It asks, *Am I open to all the possibilities life has to offer? Do I let these possibilities into my life? How is this useful to me?*

Neutral mind is meditative, intuitive, and nonattached to any specific outcome. It connects you with the guidance of your soul. It asks, *Do I allow myself to perceive and act upon inner wisdom? Does this support my purpose and vision? Is this meaningful? Is it a win-win for all?*

Relationship to Spirituality and God

The seventh chakra represents humility, vastness, and a connection to the divine.

Do you believe in God or a higher power?

If you don't believe in God, what do you believe in?

How do you bring meaning and fulfillment into your daily life?

What are your spiritual practices?

The crown chakra is the closest energy center to the infinite. When your energy moves from the first chakra to the crown chakra, you are moving toward liberation and merging with the divine. This process of liberation involves letting go of the needs of the ego for survival, security, and power, and surrendering to the will of your higher self. There comes a point in all of our lives when aspiring to achieve and accumulate wealth no longer provides fulfillment. We start to long for something more meaningful. This process requires connecting with your heart chakra to focus on what you love, where you give your time, and how you can serve the greater good, and to deepen your relationship with spirituality.

The crown chakra is the center for spiritual insight and connection with a higher purpose. It's the recognition of a higher power in the form of nature, God, Goddess, the divine, higher consciousness, and/or infinite consciousness. The yogis believe this connection with a higher power is already within us, and by acknowledging it, we experience wholeness and union. Spirituality is the way in which you express meaning and purpose, and it is your connection to the sacred—your connection with yourself, others, nature, and a higher power. Spiritualty is an individual experience. It is experiential rather than prescriptive, and it's based on love rather than on fear.

One aim of yoga is to help you become more aware of your infinite identity through spiritual practices such as meditation, time in nature, and reading books by sages and yogis. On one level, you are limited on Earth by time and space and the different roles you take on in your life. On another level, your mind is infinite and vast, and you are a creative being full of potential. Yoga reminds you that the divine is within you and you can always tune in to this energy and level of consciousness. Spirituality moves you toward expansion and vastness.

One way to understand God is as a form of energy that Generates, Organizes, and Delivers. This energy of GOD is in all things and all people. When you connect to GOD, you connect to your own power of generating, organizing, and delivering. Kundalini Yoga uses a beautiful mantra to reinforce this belief: "God and me, me and God, are one." There is no separation between you and the divine. Once this is realized, you become more aware, and you open up to an energetic support system in your life that is cocreating with you.

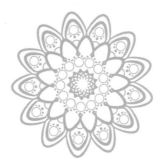

Relationship to Your Beliefs

Notice your relationship to your beliefs and how these beliefs impact your life.

What do you believe about yourself, the world, relationships, money, power, and spirituality?

When did you adopt these beliefs?

When was the last time you reflected on your beliefs and questioned them?

Beliefs are your filters for interpreting your life experiences. You learn your beliefs from your family, teachers, peers, community, and culture. In many ways, you are indoctrinated into your belief system.

As an adult, you have the power to examine and question what you believe and ask, "Does this belief expand or limit my life?"

Take time to reflect on and write down your main beliefs about health, money/finances, sexuality, power, relationships, creativity, death, spirituality, success, energy, love, God, yourself. Add any other topic that is important to you or you find yourself repeatedly struggling with in your life.

You may discover that your core negative beliefs about yourself are holding you back from manifesting what you want. Whenever you are struggling with achieving a goal, it's important to pause and look at your belief in relation to that goal.

If your goal is to take two yoga classes a week but you keep missing classes, ask yourself if you have any negative beliefs about yourself that might be sabotaging you. Beliefs may be, "I'm not flexible enough," or, "I can't commit." Replace the negative belief with one that is more affirming, such as, "I'm strong and flexible," or, "I'm disciplined." Every time you go to class, make a mental note that you are affirming this new concept of who you are. Your actions and your beliefs become aligned.

The work of the crown chakra involves continual self-reflection and self-evaluation in order for your actions to stay aligned with your values and beliefs. Common negative beliefs that sabotage us include the following:

I'm not enough. • I'm not smart enough.

I don't know enough. • I'm not safe.

I'm incomplete without a relationship. • I'm weak. • I'm not loveable.

Next time you become aware of a strong negative belief, ask yourself,

How do I know this to be true?

When did I adopt this belief?

Does this belief serve me or hinder me?

What might be a more useful/constructive belief to adopt?

The process of paying attention to your beliefs can be illuminating and healing. Take the time to update your belief system to a version that affirms and elevates who you are in the present. Liberate yourself from outdated beliefs and create more peace and alignment in your life.

Relationship to Meditation

The best practice for balancing and healing the crown chakra is meditation. Kundalini Yoga meditations use breathing techniques and mantras to cultivate a more peaceful mind.

What is your relationship with meditation?

Have you ever started a meditation practice?

If so, what helped you keep up with it, or what stopped your practice?

How can you set up a quiet place in your home where you can create a meditation sanctuary?

Meditation is the practice of calming the waves of the mind, becoming more aware, and connecting to the divine. Meditation teaches you to be still, to listen to the sensations in the body, to build a link between your body and mind, and to create a separation between you and your thoughts. The goal is not to stop thinking—that is impossible. The goal is to cultivate awareness of what you are thinking. In meditation, you learn to hover above the thoughts, observe them, and become less reactive to them. You learn that your thoughts are not always accurate, and you don't have to believe them. This is a very empowering realization. When you learn to pause before acting on any thought, you are on your way to mastering your mind and creating more peace in your life.

At some point in meditation, you will meet your edge and feel challenged. When you practice the same meditation for forty or one hundred twenty days, you will get to know all aspects of yourself. You will experience peace and bliss as well as repressed fear, guilt, shame, anger, and grief. When you can sit with all your feelings and be fully present and aware, you expand your capacity for handling discomfort. Managing intense emotions during meditation will give you better coping skills to deal with these types of emotions when they show up in daily life. When you acknowledge and accept the difficult and uncomfortable emotions within yourself, you also expand your capacity to hold space for others when they share their intense emotions. You will become less reactive and less triggered. With a regular meditation practice, you learn to be more compassionate and accepting of yourself and others, embracing the imperfections.

A daily meditation practice not only benefits you, but it can also benefit your loved ones because you become less reactive and more understanding. Start with three minutes and work toward a ten-minute meditation for forty days. A forty-day practice lets the meditation provoke your subconscious to release any thoughts and emotional patterns that hinder you. A good meditation will break your old patterns, clear the subconscious, and plant a seed for a new pattern.

Preparing for Meditation

Meditation is a personal experience, but there are a few universal suggestions that help guide the meditative experience.

- Choose a quiet space in your home or office.
- Ideally practice the meditation at the same time each day.
- Start with a three- to ten-minute practice.
- Practice the same meditation for forty days. During a forty-day cycle, you will get to know yourself, your mind, and your triggers. It's an opportunity to be with all aspects of yourself with awareness and compassion.
- Sit with a straight spine and a gentle neck lock in a chair or on the floor.
- Keep a journal and write down your experiences during the forty days. Keep the journal somewhere you can easily see it so that it reminds you to meditate.
- Be patient and kind with yourself during the practice. Your mind will wander, and there will be days when you resist the practice. That is all part of the experience. The goal is not to be a perfect meditator, but to show up and meditate every day.
- Start your forty-day cycle with a friend to keep each other motivated and accountable.

- Be flexible with your practice. Some days you may have to practice in your car or at the office. Let go of any critical judgments when things don't go according to plan. Have fun with the practice.

Benefits of Meditation

- Focuses the wandering mind
- Reduces stress and anxiety
- Cultivates more clarity and focus
- Provides reprieve from stressors of daily life
- Improves willpower and self-control
- Develops self-awareness
- Encourages quality time with yourself to recognize and connect with your true nature
- Allows you to receive guidance from your higher self
- Expands your capacity for discomfort as you face the challenges of maintaining a daily practice
- Opens you up to a deeper relationship with the divine

Relationship to Your Brain

Consider these questions:

What are your recurring worries and stressors?

How often do you notice experiencing the fight, flight, or freeze response in a given day?

How does this feel in your body?

How often do you pause and notice the good around you?

How does this feel in your body?

Research has established that the brain physically changes based on your experiences and thought patterns. If you are continually focusing on criticism, worry, and stress, this property, known as neuroplasticity, causes your brain to become increasingly reactive and prone to anxiety and fear. If, on the other hand, you focus your mind on positive events and experiences, your brain becomes more optimistic and resilient.

In his book *Hardwiring Happiness*, Dr. Rick Hanson describes how our brains are wired to a default setting that notices danger and threatening situations much more than positive situations and experiences. He explains that our ancestors' survival depended on what is now called the "negativity bias" and our brain's ability to detect danger.[12] This negativity bias doesn't serve us as well as it served our ancestors because most of us are no longer facing life-threating dangers in our daily lives. Yet, it seems that we routinely overestimate the threats in our lives while underestimating the opportunities and resources.

Physiologically, it goes like this: first, whenever we perceive a threat, the fear center in our brain, called the amygdala, gets triggered. Next, the amygdala signals the hypothalamus to release adrenaline, cortisol, norepinephrine, and other stress hormones into the blood. Then, we either freeze, fight, or flee from the perceived threat. Even after the perceived threat has passed, our bodies are still flooded throughout the day with these hormones that overtax and deplete the nervous system.

Your Brain's Response to Threat

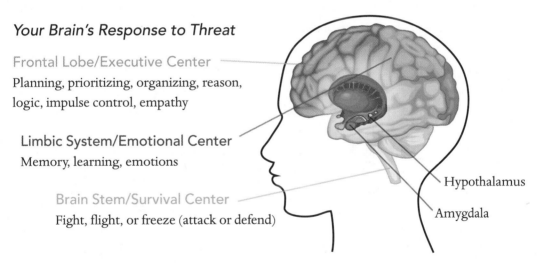

Frontal Lobe/Executive Center
Planning, prioritizing, organizing, reason, logic, impulse control, empathy

Limbic System/Emotional Center
Memory, learning, emotions

Brain Stem/Survival Center
Fight, flight, or freeze (attack or defend)

Hypothalamus

Amygdala

Self-awareness, meditation, and consciously looking for the good experiences in your life can retrain your brain and your mind toward noticing more positive experiences and

12. Hanson, *Hardwiring Happiness*, 10–31.

fewer negative ones. This shift will decrease the number of times your amygdala gets triggered and sends you into overdrive. Research has shown that regular meditators have more gray matter in their frontal cortex, which is the part of the brain responsible for higher-order thinking, planning ahead, working toward goals, and making decisions. Specific parts of the frontal cortex can talk down the amygdala so it's not consistently pushing the alarm button. We can train the amygdala to stop firing off the alarm bell as often as it does to perceived threats.

A regular meditation practice increases your awareness, and your awareness helps you hit the pause button before reacting to fear and danger. Instead of reacting, self-awareness helps you respond with a few deep breaths so that you can ask yourself, "Am I really in danger at this moment? Can I handle this situation without flooding my system with stress hormones? What resources are available to help me?" Several times a day, pause for a moment and look for the good or recall a happy memory. Continue to visualize it, and connect with the sensations it evokes in your body for thirty seconds to one minute. Making this simple exercise a daily habit retrains your brain toward happiness rather than distress.

Discover how your thoughts relate to your chakras.
What are you thinking about?

Chakra One: Survival, fear, safety, finances, health, and home

Chakra Two: Desires, passions, feelings, sexuality, worrying, longing for something

Chakra Three: Activity, your to-do list, what you are accomplishing and getting done

Chakra Four: Relationships, love, social interactions, and compassion

Chakra Five: Communication, conversation, mental dialogue, arguing, writing, and thinking about what you want to say

Chakra Six: Imagining, fantasizing, daydreaming, remembering, being out of present time

Chakra Seven: Thinking, analyzing, problem-solving, spiritual practices, prayer, meditating

Where has your mind been resting?

How much time do you spend in each of the areas associated with each chakra? Is there one chakra that dominates your thinking more than the others? If so, how do these thought patterns influence your brain and your outlook on life? What would you like to change in your thought patterns?

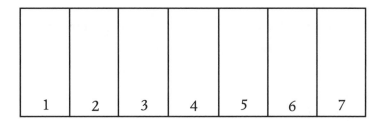

| 1 | 2 | 3 | 4 | 5 | 6 | 7 |

Using the corresponding chakra color, fill in each rectangle to indicate the amount of time you focus on the issues associated with that chakra. How high does each chakra rise?

Relationship to Sleep

Sleep is a biological necessity we need to survive. Experts recommend adults get seven to eight hours of sleep each night.

On average, how many hours of sleep do you get?

Do you feel rested when you wake up in the morning?

What is your routine to wind down in the evening and get ready for bed?

Sleep is a vital element in keeping the crown chakra healthy and balanced. Lack of sleep affects your energy, mood, and memory. Research has shown that sleep deprivation can have severe consequences for your overall health and can lead to diabetes, increased body aches and pains, and reduced immune function.

Ideally you want to get seven to eight hours of restful sleep each night. A daily yoga and meditation practice as well as lifestyle changes can improve your sleep. Kundalini Yoga meditations are said to stimulate the pineal gland, located in the middle of the brain, which secretes melatonin, a hormone that may help regulate sleep.

Tips for better sleep[13]

- Stick to a sleep schedule by going to bed at the same time every day.
- Get outside in natural sunlight for at least thirty minutes every day.
- Consume any caffeine and/or nicotine before noon.
- Avoid alcoholic drinks and large meals before bed.
- If you nap, do so before 3:00 p.m.
- Unplug from work and wind down before getting into bed.
- Take a hot shower or bath before bed.
- Start to dim the lights a few hours before bed.
- Keep the bedroom dark and the temperature around 65°F.
- Keep your bedroom gadget-free.

Relationship to Attachment

Attachment is the desire to keep control or to hold on to things, people, and experiences. But this is in direct conflict with the cycle of life because nothing stays the same; change is the only constant in life.

What are you most attached to in your life?

How attached are you to outcomes in your life?

How do you react when you don't get what you want?

What are you ready to let go of that is no longer serving you?

One of the main challenges to overcome at the crown chakra is letting go of our need or desire to possess, grasp, and hold on to possessions, people, beliefs, and habits. Attachment confines you to time and place and limits your possibilities as you fixate on one thing. Attachment is helpful in managing day-to-day life from the lower chakras, as it helps you get things done and form lasting relationships. This same quality can become

---

13. Matthew Walker, *Why We Sleep: Unlocking The Power of Sleep and Dreams* (New York: Scribner, 2017), 3–78.

an obstacle in the crown chakra because it can limit your awareness and hinder your growth to embrace uncertainty. An open and balanced crown chakra allows you to live and love fully without any attachment to the outcome of your actions.

Few of us attain this level of awareness in daily life. A mantra for the crown chakra is, "Let thy will be done." This attitude takes a great deal of trust in the universe and surrendering of the individual ego to merge with the divine. Trusting in the process of life, you allow things, people, and experiences to come and go without attachment. It helps to see life from the vantage point of the cosmos in the most expansive way possible—rather than from the details and emotional dramas of daily life—and to cultivate a deep level of humility to serve others. Next time you are in the grips of attachment, ask yourself, "What is the meaning and purpose of this situation? How am I learning and growing? How am I helping others?"

Notice what you are most attached to in your life. How much energy do you exert on keeping the attachments in your life? Does this seem like a good use of your energy? Attachment creates suffering when it drains your energy and you can't think about anything else. It limits your capacity to see the bigger picture and to value what is within you more than what is outside of you. The crown chakra teaches us to let go and to surrender to the wisdom of the universe—to surrender to the unknown.

The practice of nonattachment throughout life can prepare us to let go during death. If we condition the mind to let go freely and with ease throughout life, we can let go of our last breath with grace. If we have taken risks during life and allowed room for uncertainty, we can face the unknown of the afterlife. When I become too attached in my life, I sit with it for a few minutes, feel the attachment in my body, and notice all the emotions that arise. Then I imagine that I'm a spiritual being visiting this planet to have a human experience with all of its ups and downs and that I'm here for a short time to have a rich and full experience. This particular attachment is teaching me something, and sometimes these teachings are painful. The most painful of these experiences is the death of loved ones because I become so attached to missing their physical form in my life. Over time, I let go of the attachment to the particular form that person took, and I start to see them in nature and to feel them in my heart. With awareness and love, I open up to a deeper understanding of death and the connection between myself and loved ones. Attachment is an opportunity to go deeper within and gain a richer understanding of life.

Kundalini Meditation to Sleep, Live, and Love Better

The best time to practice this meditation is at night before bed, but it can be practiced any time of the day. It is said that if it is practiced regularly, sleep will be deep and relaxed, and the nerves will regenerate. After a few months, the rhythm of your breath as you sleep will be subconsciously regulated in the rhythm of the mantra. You will think clearer, work smarter, and love better.

Posture: Sit in any comfortable posture with the spine straight. Place the hands in the lap, palms up, with the right hand over the left. The thumbs are together and point forward.

Eye Focus: Focus the eyes on the tip of the nose, with the eyelids nine-tenths closed.

Breath and Mantra: Inhale in four equal parts, mentally vibrating the mantra *Sa-Ta-Na-Ma*. Hold the breath, vibrating the mantra four times for a total of sixteen beats. Exhale in two equal strokes, projecting mentally *Wahe Guru*.

Time: Practice for five to thirty minutes.

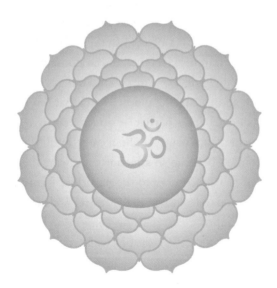

Questions

1. Describe your relationship with your mind.

2. What is your level of self-awareness?

3. What does spirituality mean to you? What portion of your life is spent in the practice of spirituality?

4. When was the last time you reflected on your beliefs? In what ways do you think your beliefs impact your life?

5. What do you think is the meaning of life?

_____

_____

_____

_____

_____

_____

_____

_____

_____

_____

_____

_____

_____

_____

_____

Crown Chakra Short Practice

One-Minute Breath

Sit in easy pose with a straight spine. Inhale for twenty seconds, hold for twenty seconds, exhale for twenty seconds. Start with five to ten seconds if twenty seconds is challenging. Make sure all three segments of the breath are equal in length.

> *Benefits:* Optimized cooperation between the brain hemispheres; calming of anxiety, fear, and worry. Cultivates intuition and whole-brain functioning.

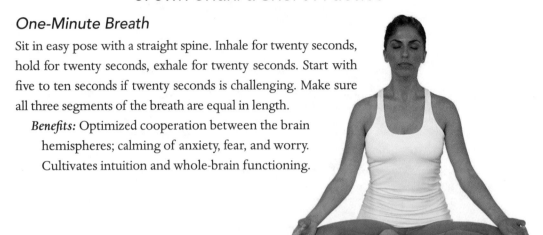

Triangle Pose

Begin in table pose with the wrists under the shoulders and hips over the knees. Push into the hands and feet and lift the body into a triangle. Lengthen the spine, draw the shoulder blades toward each other, relax the head, push the legs away from you, and press the heels toward the earth. Breathe long and deep. Hold for two to three minutes.

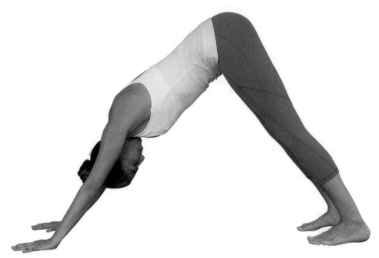

> *Benefits:* Increases circulation to the face and head. Increases mental clarity and improves complexion. Strengthens the nervous system.

Rabbit Pose

Kneel in rock pose. Reach behind and grasp your heels, thumbs on the outside of the feet, heels resting securely in your palms. Inhale, and on the exhale, lower the upper torso, tucking your chin toward your chest, and let the crown of your head rest on the floor. Grasp the heels tighter and raise your hips until your arms are straight. Pull on your heels. Use the strength of your arms to make sure your weight is not on your head or neck. Hold for one minute, and then lower hips to slowly return to rock pose.

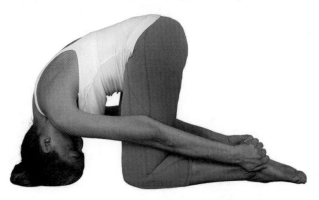

Benefits: Increases the flow of energy along the sushumna; brings increased energy and circulation to the crown chakra; stimulates and brings a fresh supply of blood to the brain, pituitary, thyroid, and parathyroid glands.

Silent Meditation

Sit in easy pose with hands in gyan mudra. Close the eyes and focus them upward on the crown chakra. Breathe long and deep. Be still and silent. Continue for three to eleven minutes.

Benefits: Calms and clears the mind and slows respiration and heart rate.

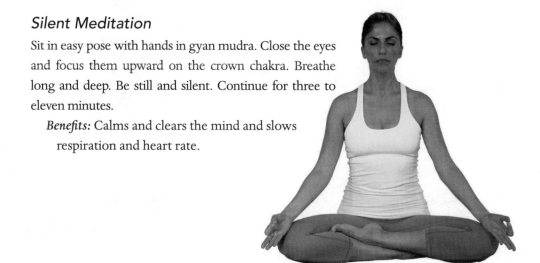

Crown Chakra Warm-Ups

Practice each pose for one to two minutes.

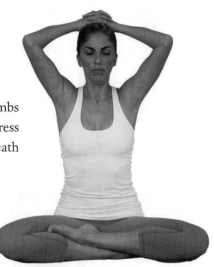

1. Easy Pose with Breath of Fire

Sit in easy pose, interlace the fingers with the thumbs
touching, and let the hands rest on top of the head. Press
the tongue against the roof of the mouth. Begin breath
of fire.

2. Spinal Flex

Sit in easy pose and bring the arms out to the sides. Inhale, extend the spine forward,
and stretch the arms back. Exhale, push the spine back, and wrap the arms around the
shoulders.

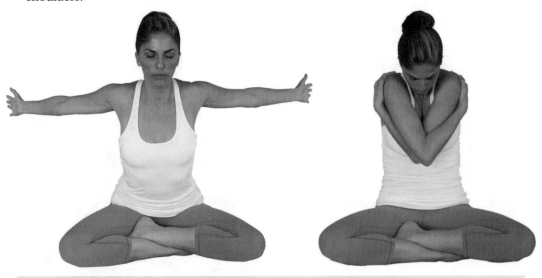

3. Spinal Twist

Sit in easy pose and bring the hands to the shoulders with the fingers in front and the thumbs in back. Inhale and twist to the left and exhale to twist to the right.

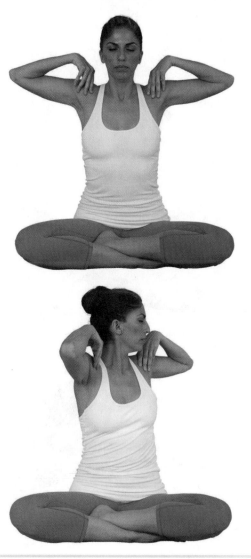

4. Wide Leg Forward Fold

Open the legs wide. Inhale and stretch the arms overhead. Exhale and turn to the left, hinging from the hips, and reach forward. Inhale to the center and exhale to the right, hinging from the hips and reaching forward.

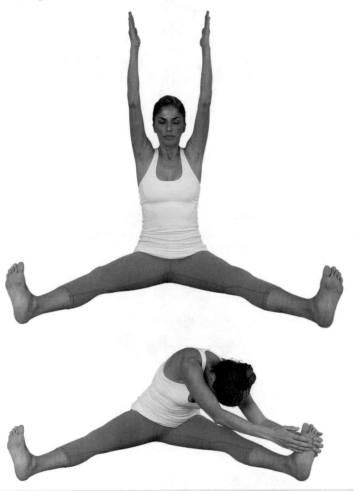

5. *Sitting Forward Fold*

Bring the legs together and flex the toes toward the head. Inhale and stretch both arms up. Exhale and reach for the toes. Wrap the thumb and fingers around the big toes and squeeze. Inhale and lengthen the spine up and exhale as you lower down toward the legs. Hold with long, deep breaths.

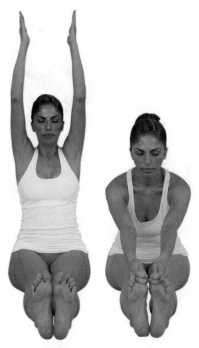

6. Cat Cow

Come onto all fours and place the wrists under the shoulders and the knees under the hips. Make sure there is space between the knees. Inhale and drop the spine down and lift the head up. Exhale and round the spine upward and drop the head down. Continue at your own pace.

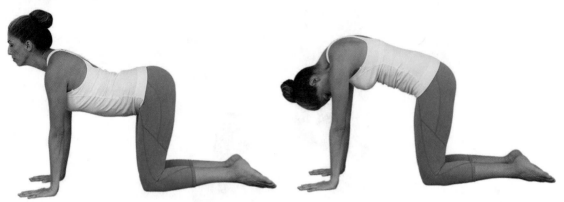

7. Triangle Pose

Begin in table pose with the wrists under the shoulders and the hips over the knees. Push into the hands and feet and lift the body into a triangle. Lengthen the spine, draw the shoulder blades toward each other, relax the head, push the legs away from you, and press the heels toward the earth. Breathe long and deep.

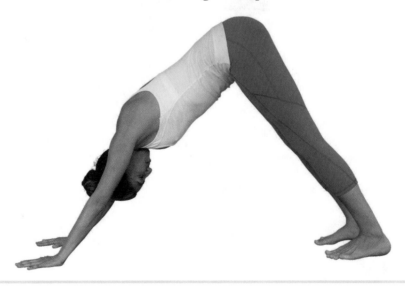

Sat Kriya Variation to Merge with the Infinite

This kriya elevates your body, mind, and spirit so that you can merge with the infinite energy. Boundaries fall away, and you become aware of your interconnection to all things.

Posture

Sit in easy pose.

Mudra

Raise the right arm straight up. The palm is open and faces toward the left. The fingers of the right hand are spread open. The right shoulder is slightly lifted as you fully extend the arm upward. The left arm rests over the left knee.

Eye Focus

Eyes are closed.

Mantra

Chant *Sat Nam* in a constant rhythm, about eight times per ten seconds. Chant *Sat* from the navel, pulling the navel point all the way in toward the spine. On *Nam*, relax the belly.

Time

Practice for five to thirty minutes.

To end

Inhale deeply, suspend the breath as you squeeze the muscles tightly, and stretch the right arm up. Concentrate on the flow of energy along the entire length of the spine and through the crown chakra. Exhale powerfully. Repeat this sequence two more times.

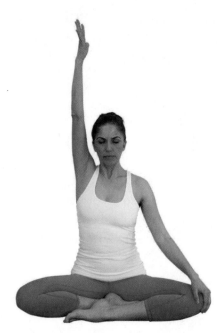

Relax *for eleven to fifteen minutes*

Rest on your back with the legs straight and the feet splayed out to the sides. Make sure you are warm and comfortable as you begin this relaxation. Soften the ankles, calves, and shins and let the thighs melt into the floor. Visualize a beautiful violet light around your entire body balancing your crown chakra. Allow your breath to find its own natural rhythm while softening the navel area. Relax the chest, shoulders, arms, and hands. Soften the muscles in the neck and throat. Let your entire face soften. Continue to see a spiraling violet light around your head, showering you with healing energy and restoring your connection with the divine.

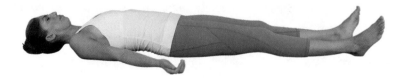

Meditation for the Neutral Mind

This meditation cultivates awareness and a deeper connection to your higher self and your inner light. A regular practice will keep you calm, clearheaded, and centered within yourself, even when life is stressful and challenging.

Posture

Sit in easy pose with the spine straight.

Mudra

Place both hands in the lap with the palms facing up. Rest the right hand in the left. The thumb tips may or may not touch.

Eye Focus

Focus at the brow point. Remove all tension from every part of the body. Imagine seeing yourself sitting peacefully and full of radiance. Then gradually let your energy collect like a flow at the brow point.

Mantra

Wha Hay Guru

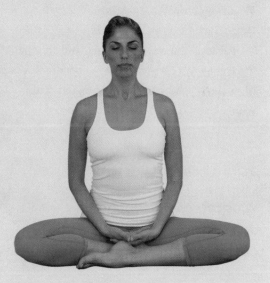

This mantra expresses the indescribable experience of going from darkness to light—from ignorance to true understanding. It calls on the higher self to keep going steadily through all barriers.

Breath

Natural breathing.

Time

Practice for ten to thirty minutes.

Meditation for Letting Go

This meditation helps you let go of attachments to the finite self and open up to grace and acceptance during times of change and transition. With practice, it can give you the capacity to embody a divine personality and become creative and fearless.

Posture
Sit in easy pose with a light Jalandhar bandha (neck lock).

Eye Focus
Focus at the brow point.

Mudra
Let the hands rest in the lap, right hand in the left palm, or just sit with both hands in gyan mudra. Become completely still, physically and mentally, like a calm ocean. Listen to the chant for a minute. Feel its rhythm in every cell. Then join in the mantra.

Mantra
Pavan Pavan Pavan Pavan Para Paraa,
Pavan Guroo Pavan Guru,
Wha-Hay Guru Wha-Hay Guru,
Pavan Guru

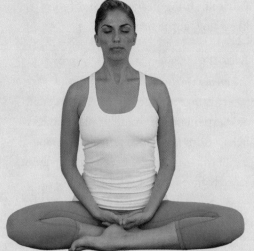

    Pavan is the air, the breath, and the life force energy. This mantra increases the flow of prana so that you feel contained within yourself and can let go when necessary.

Time
Practice for ten to thirty minutes.

Music Recommendations
Sat Purkh, *The Guru Within*
Guru Shabd Singh Khalsa, *Pavan, Pavan*

Part 5
Expanding on the Chakras

Unlike other yoga traditions, Kundalini Yoga includes the aura as the eighth chakra. The aura is an electromagnetic field that surrounds the body and projects the energy of the other chakras. A person with a strong aura exudes charisma, kindness, compassion, and uplifting energy. We are drawn to people with strong auras and feel good in their presence. In the following chapter, you will find practices for building a strong, radiant aura.

You will also find a chapter that includes a yoga set and meditations to keep all the chakras balanced and your aura bright. Whether or not you have explored the other sets in this book, you can jump to this chapter at any point in your journey. Turn to this practice whenever you feel the need for integration, and invite more harmony as you balance all the chakras in unison.

Be the light.

Chapter 9
THE AURA (8th Chakra)

Translation: Radiance

Main Issues: Protection, projection, charisma, sensitivity

Element: None

Location: Electromagnetic field surrounding the physical body

Color: White

Goals: To have an uplifting presence and to feel safe and secure

Balanced Energy

- Grounded
- Feeling safe and protected
- Charismatic
- Ability to filter out negative influences
- Connected to others without merging with their energy
- Radiant

Deficient Energy

- Paranoid
- Vulnerable
- Easily influenced by others
- Inability to trust
- Drained after social interactions
- Internalizing other people's feelings as their own

Healing Practices

Meditation

Positive thinking

All breathing exercises

Wear white clothing

Drink lots of water

Take Epsom salt baths

Shower at the end of the day

Sing joyously

Affirmations

I am light and I am bright.

I am kind and compassionate.

My life force energy is strong and radiant.

My presence inspires and uplifts.

I trust in myself and I trust in the divine.

I'm connected to heaven and Earth.

The Aura and Your Chakras

> Notice your sense of integration and radiance.
>
> *How do you connect with the energy of your aura?*
>
> *Can you tell when your aura feels strong and when it feels weak?*

Many yoga traditions end with the crown chakra, but Kundalini Yoga includes the aura as the eighth chakra. The eighth chakra represents radiance, the electromagnetic field, and protection. The aura is distributed around the body like an egg shape or oval cocoon and contains your life force energy. The aura changes in color, brightness, and size depending on your health, your thoughts, and your feelings.

The eighth chakra combines the effects of the other chakras and is a reflection of your inner health and well-being. When all the chakras are balanced and integrated, the aura fully radiates, protects you from negative influences, and projects your energy out. The aura delivers and receives messages to and from the other chakras.

The Layers of Your Aura[14]

Visualize your aura as having seven layers of subtle energy that correspond to the characteristics of the seven chakras. The layers of the aura can have different frequencies, and often one layer dominates in energy over the others.

- *Connection*
- *Intuition*
- *Truth*
- *Love*
- *Energy*
- *Emotions*
- *Instinct*

---

14. Cyndi Dale, *Energetic Boundaries: How to Stay Protected and Connected in Work, Love, and Life* (Boulder, CO: Sounds True, 2011), 5–45.

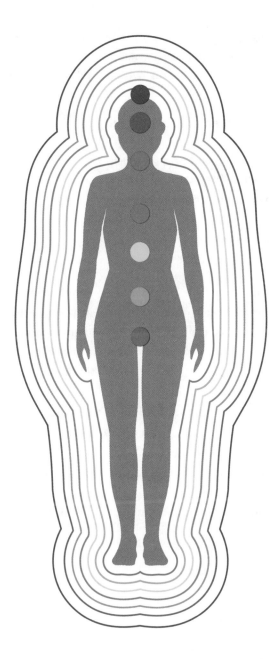

The seventh layer is your connection to spirituality. The color is violet.

The sixth layer relates to intuition and the connection to the subtle realms. The color is indigo.

The fifth layer relates to your creative expression and communication. The color is blue.

The fourth layer is related to your heart and emotions and the interactions you have in your main relationships. The color is green.

The third layer shows how you interact with your environment and society and your expression of personal power. The color is yellow.

The second layer relates to emotional safety and well-being. The color is orange.

The first layer is closest to the body and represents your health. This layer is the anchor to the earth. The color is red.

Relationship to Your Immediate Environment

> Take a moment and think about the people in your life who energize you and those who drain your energy. Also notice which environments balance your energy and which make you feel out of balance.
>
> *How much personal space do you need to feel safe and secure?*
>
> *What environments make you feel vibrant and energized, and which ones make you feel lethargic, dull, and weak?*
>
> *How susceptible are you to taking on other people's feelings and thoughts?*
>
> *What helps you maintain clear boundaries?*

The aura is an energy field around the body, and the boundary between your personal energy and the energy of others. The aura lets you know what is happening in the present moment. It contains and filters thoughts, feelings, attitudes, and interactions between you and your environment. The aura is an early warning system that detects negative energy and disturbances in your environment. Disease in the physical, emotional, and mental bodies is often experienced in the aura first.

The aura sends out and receives your energy, thoughts, and emotions to and from the world. If the aura holds on to these messages for too long, it can overload your system. This overload can lead to incessant mental chatter, feeling crowded or claustrophobic, and/or sensing a lack of personal space. Merging with other people's energy creates an aura of lowered vitality and can lead to illness.

To strengthen your aura, practice visualizing these images around your physical body:

- A clear crystal sphere
- A forest of trees
- A pink bubble
- A waterfall
- Mirrors
- Thick golden light

Relationship to Your Radiance

Your radiance is your magnetic attraction and ability to influence and succeed. Your radiance is your beauty and brightness, and it shines through in your aura.

Who do you know who has a magnetic presence?
What brings out your light and your radiance?
Are you comfortable being in the spotlight, or do you shy away from attention?

When you feel healthy, grounded, and confident, your aura will be strong and radiant. It will expand in all directions and show strong colors and vibrations. When the aura is balanced, it creates a sense of presence and charisma. It attracts resources to you and deflects negativity. When the aura is strong, it acts as a container for your life force energy, and your presence alone is enough to influence any situation.

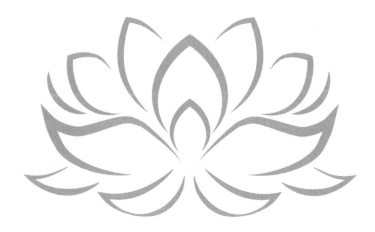

Visualizations to Expand and Strengthen the Aura

Sit in easy pose and bring your focus inward. Begin to mentally chant, *I am Bright and I am Light*. After practicing this mantra for three minutes, notice the sensations and feelings that it evokes. Focus on these feelings and fill the room with your energy and presence. Visualize expanding your light and your aura to the four corners of the room.

Several times during the day, notice the energy around your body and sense how far your aura extends. Sense the energy in the back, to the sides, and in front of you. Visualize a healing waterfall of life force energy showering you and cleansing your aura, and visualize your aura flowing down into the grounding energy of the earth.

Practice for three to five minutes.

Questions

1. Do you feel safe in the world?

2. How does your energy uplift and inspire others?

3. In the presence of other people, are you more aware of your own thoughts and feelings or of theirs?

4. Do you tend to give in to peer pressure or hold your ground?

5. What in your life makes you feel elevated and expansive?

6. Do you see yourself as radiant and charismatic?

_____

_____

_____

_____

_____

_____

_____

_____

Aura Short Practice

Auric Sweep

Stand with the feet hip-distance apart. Inhale, sweep your arms toward the sky, and bring the palms together. Exhale and let the arms float back down to the sides of your legs. Continue the movement for three minutes, then sit for a moment and assess your aura and its vastness.

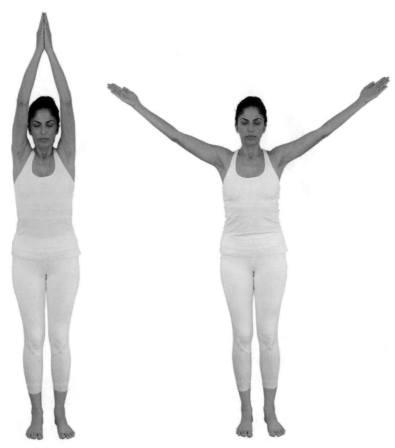

Benefits: Recharges your aura and gives you radiance.

Triangle Pose

Begin in table pose with the wrists directly under the shoulders and the hips directly over the knees. Push into the hands and feet and lift the body into a triangle. Lengthen the spine, draw the shoulder blades toward each other, relax the head, push the legs away from you, and press the heels toward the earth. Breathe long and deep. Hold for one to two minutes.

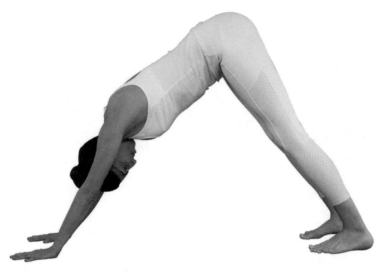

Benefits: Strengthens the nervous system so you can have nerves of steel, aids digestion, and stretches and strengthens all your major muscles.

Ego Eradicator

Sit in easy pose and apply neck lock. Curl the fingers in toward the palms and stretch the thumbs up. Lift your arms up to 60 degrees and stretch the thumbs back, pointing them toward each other. Eyes are closed and focused at the brow point. Begin breath of fire. Hold for two to three minutes.

Benefits: Strengthens the aura / electro-magnetic field. The ego is transformed and balanced and the heart chakra is expanded.

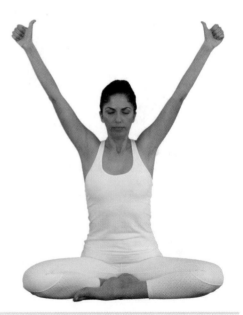

Meditation for Radiance and Ease

Sit in easy pose with a straight spine. The hands are resting in the lap. Palms face up, one resting on top of the other. It doesn't matter which hand is on top. Point the thumbs away from the body and join them at their tips.Let yourself totally relax and be comfortable throughout the meditation. Breathe naturally.

Close the eyes and mentally look around you. Tune in to the aura and feel that you are part of Mother Nature. Feel that you are a star in the vastness and the beauty of the blue sky. Perceive your own radiance. Begin with three minutes and slowly build up to ten minutes.

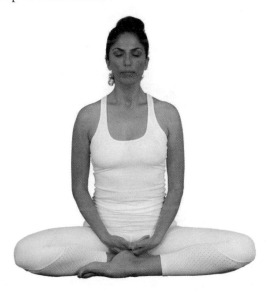

Aura Warm-Ups

Practice each pose for one to two minutes.

1. Spinal Flex with the Arms

Sit in easy pose. Bring your arms out to the sides, inhale and extend the spine forward, and stretch the arms behind you. Exhale and stretch the spine back and bring opposite hands to opposite shoulders.

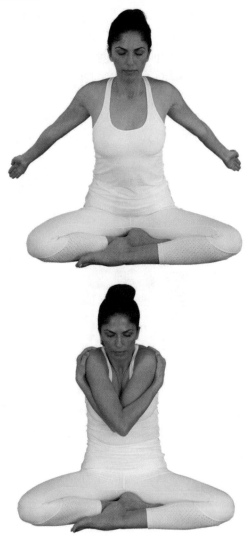

2. Spinal Twist

Place your hands on your shoulders with fingertips in the front and thumbs in the back. Inhale and twist to the left. Exhale and twist to the right.

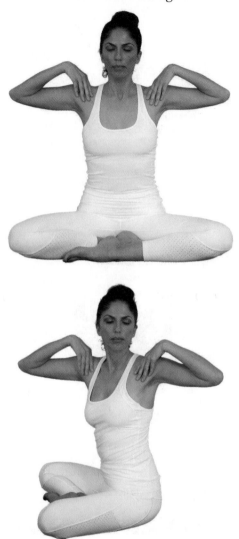

3. Elbow Raises

Keep the hands on the shoulders, inhale, and bring the elbows up toward the ceiling. Exhale and lower them to shoulder height.

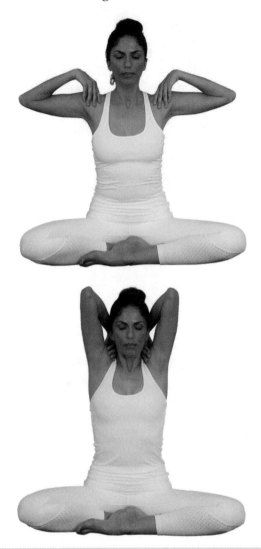

4. High Cobra Pose to Triangle Pose

Begin in table pose with the wrists directly under the shoulders and the hips directly over the knees. Push into the hands and feet and lift the body into a triangle pose. Inhale and come into a high cobra with the hips off the floor and the shoulders down and away from the ears. Exhale and press back into triangle pose. Continue alternating between the two poses.

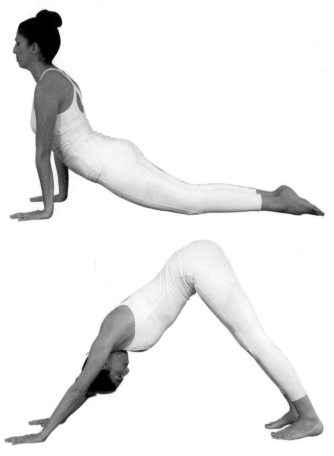

5. Aura Sweep with Prayer Pose

Stand with the feet hip-distance apart. Inhale, and raise the arms up until the palms touch. Exhale and lower the hands to prayer pose. Visualize a golden light around you as you sweep the arms up and back down. Visualize a strong, balanced aura.

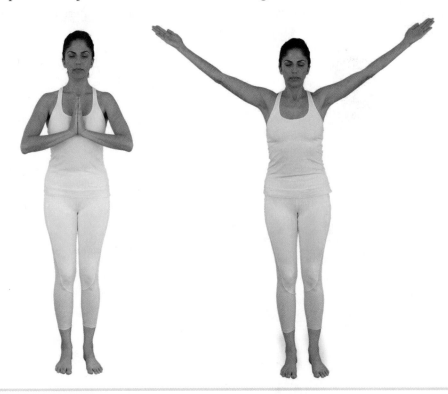

6. Aura Sweep with Forward Fold

Inhale and raise the arms overhead with the palms facing up. Exhale as you fold forward from the hips and sweep the arms down and behind the legs. Inhale backup. Visualize clearing the energy in front of and behind you.

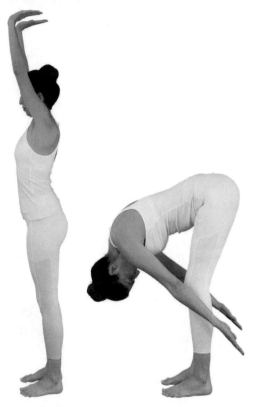

Focus on the mantra, *"I am Bright and I am Light."*

7. Goddess Pose

Stand with the legs wide apart and the feet pointing out. Bend the knees until the thighs are parallel to the floor. Stretch the arms out to the sides at shoulder height with the palms facing forward. Press the feet into the earth, engage the muscles in the legs, and lengthen the spine. Breathe long and deep.

8. Archer Pose

Stand with your legs wide apart (two to three feet) and your feet parallel to each other. Turn the right foot 90 degrees and bend the knee over the ankle so that the thigh is parallel to the floor. Back left foot is at a 45-degree angle. Lengthen the spine and bring the arms up to shoulder height. Curl the fingers of both hands and stretch the thumbs up. Bend the left elbow and turn to face the right thumb. Focus on the tip of the right thumb with the eyes open. Continue with long, deep breathing. Switch sides.

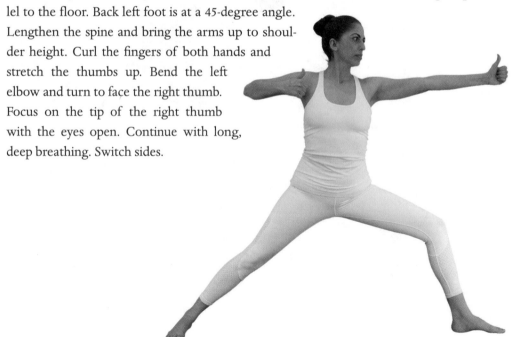

Kriya for the Aura

This is a powerful kriya for developing your aura. It strengthens the body by cultivating strength and stamina, helps you release negative energy, and brightens your aura.

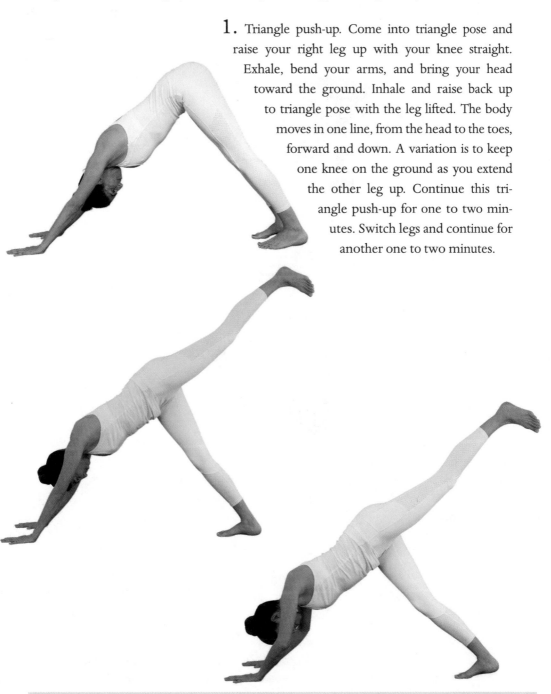

1. Triangle push-up. Come into triangle pose and raise your right leg up with your knee straight. Exhale, bend your arms, and bring your head toward the ground. Inhale and raise back up to triangle pose with the leg lifted. The body moves in one line, from the head to the toes, forward and down. A variation is to keep one knee on the ground as you extend the other leg up. Continue this triangle push-up for one to two minutes. Switch legs and continue for another one to two minutes.

2. Extend your left hand forward as if grasping a pole. The palm faces to the right. Cross the right hand beneath the left, palm down. Drop the thumb so that the palm faces the right. Grasp the left hand (the right fingers over the left hand) and lock the thumbs. Inhale and raise the arms to 60 degrees. Exhale and bring the arms down to shoulder level. Keep the elbows straight. Continue for two to three minutes. To end, inhale and stretch the arms up. Relax.

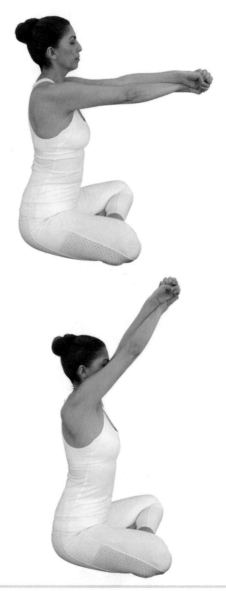

3. Bring your arms out in front with your hands at the level of the face and your palms facing each other, six inches apart. As you inhale, swing the arms down and back. Exhale and bring them forward to the original position. Continue for two to three minutes with deep, rhythmic breaths.

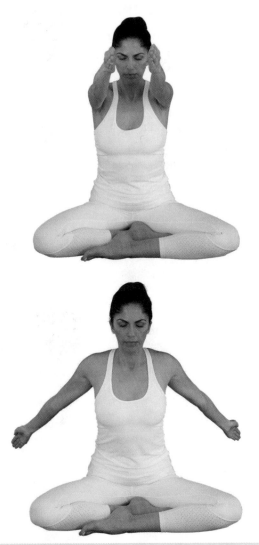

Meditation for Projection and Protection

This mantra surrounds the magnetic field with protective light and opens the heart center.

Posture

Sit in an easy pose with a light neck lock.

Mudra

Inhale at the heart chakra to begin. Chant the first line of the mantra as the arms move up and out to a 45-degree angle. Inhale and bring the hands back to the heart chakra. Exhale and chant the second line of the mantra. Continue in the same way for each line of the mantra. Inhale each time the hands return to the heart chakra. Project your mind to infinity as you chant.

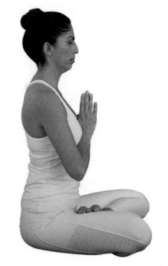

Mantra

Aad Guray Nameh
(I bow to the primal wisdom)
Jugad Guray Nameh (I bow to the wisdom through the ages)
Sat Guray Nameh (I bow to the true wisdom)
Siri Guru Devay Nameh
(I bow to the great unseen wisdom)

Time

Practice for five to thirty minutes.

To End

Inhale deeply and relax.

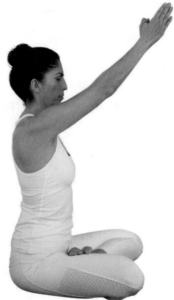

Music Recommendations

Gurunam Singh, *Touch Every Heart: Meditations for Transformation*
Snatum Kaur, *Celebrate Peace*

Meditation for Trust

This meditation builds trust so that you feel supported and guided by the infinite. It also strengthens the aura so that you can meet the challenges in your life and stay steady.

Posture

Sit in easy pose with a straight spine.

Mudra

Using your arms, create an arch over your head with the palms facing down. If you want to connect with your masculine energy, place the right palm on top of the left. If you want to connect with your feminine energy, place the left palm on top of the right. Thumb tips are together with the thumbs pointing away from you. Arms are slightly bent at the elbows.

Eye Focus

The eyes are open slightly and look down toward the upper lip.

Mantra

Wahe Guru (indescribable ecstasy)

Begin to whisper the mantra. Be very precise with pronouncing the words with your lips and tongue. Whisper so that *Guru* is almost inaudible. Each repetition lasts about two and a half seconds.

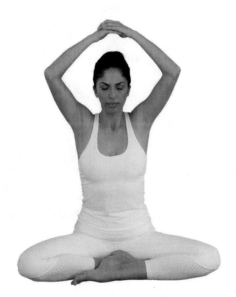

Time

Continue for five to thirty minutes.

To End

Inhale deeply and exhale. Relax.

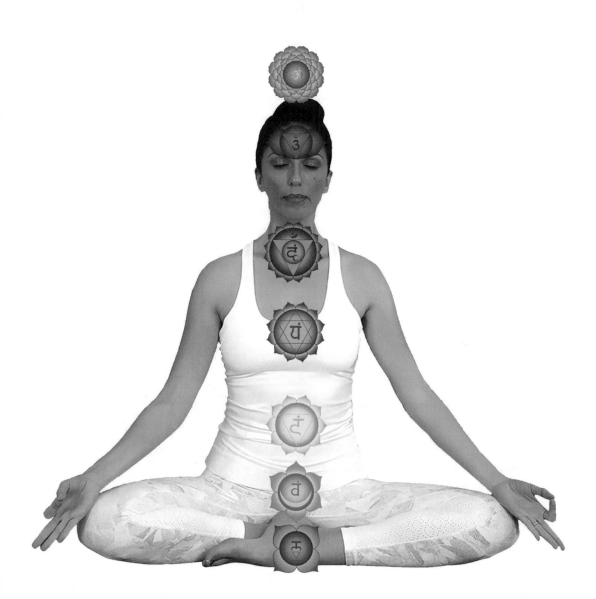

Chapter 10
Energize and Balance the Chakras

Sat Kriya for the chakras is a powerful yoga set to balance the energies in all your chakras. The set includes one pose with a specific mudra and visualization for each chakra so that all your chakras receive an energetic tune-up. You are chanting the mantra, Sat Nam, in each pose to focus the mind; to balance the elements of earth, water, fire, air, and ether; and to connect more deeply with the truth of your soul.

Sat Kriya strengthens the nervous system, calms emotions, channels creative and sexual energy, and releases old patterns that no longer serve you. Practice this yoga once a week or whenever your chakras need a reset.

Warm-Ups to Energize and Balance the Chakras

Practice each pose for one to two minutes.

1. Bridge Pose

Keep the knees bent with feet parallel and hip-distance apart. Position the heels near the buttocks. Arms reach down to grab the ankles or rest on the floor with palms down. Inhale and push the feet down into the ground while lifting the thighs toward the ceiling. Walk the shoulder blades toward one another. Hold the pose with long, deep breathing, and continue to lift a little higher with each inhalation.

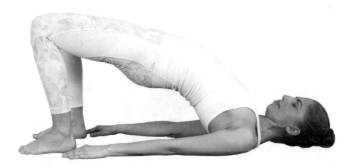

2. Drop Knees Side to Side

Stay on your back with the knees bent and the feet hip-distance apart. Slowly start to drop the knees side to side as slowly as you can so you can feel the sensations in your hips.

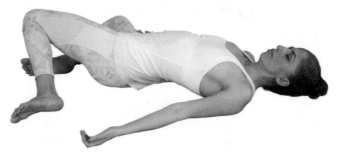

3. Bridge Pose with Hip Opener

Stay on your back and bring the soles of your feet together. Lift the hips off the floor halfway up. Hold with long, deep breaths.

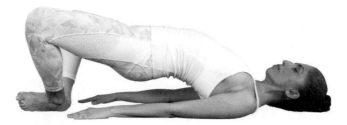

4. Cat Cow

Come onto all fours and place the wrists under the shoulders and the knees under the hips. Make sure there is space between the knees. Inhale and drop the spine down and lift the head up. Exhale and round the spine upward and drop the head down. Continue at your own pace.

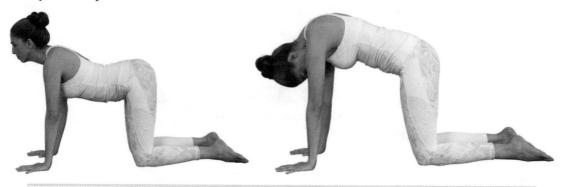

5. Triangle Pose

Begin in table pose with the wrists under the shoulders and the hips over the knees. Push into the hands and feet and lift the body into a triangle. Lengthen the spine, draw the shoulder blades toward one another, relax the head, push the legs away, and press the heels toward the earth. Breathe long and deep.

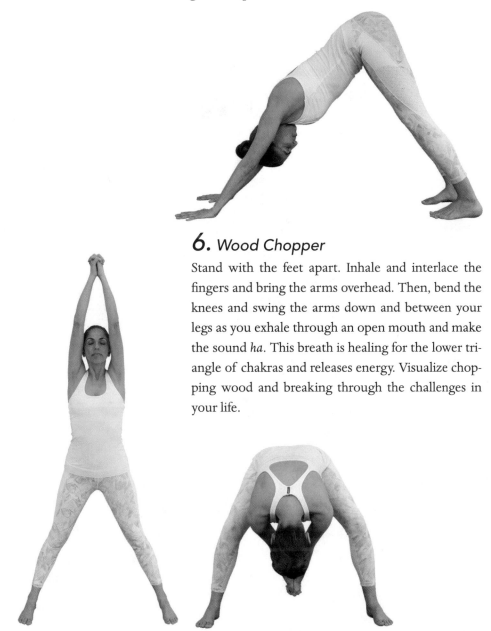

6. Wood Chopper

Stand with the feet apart. Inhale and interlace the fingers and bring the arms overhead. Then, bend the knees and swing the arms down and between your legs as you exhale through an open mouth and make the sound *ha*. This breath is healing for the lower triangle of chakras and releases energy. Visualize chopping wood and breaking through the challenges in your life.

7. Backbend with Breath of Fire

Stand with the feet together or hip-distance apart and engage your navel point. Bring the arms together over your head, clasp the hands, and point the index finger up toward the ceiling. Gently press the hips forward and lift the chest up and lean back as far as is comfortable for you. Begin breath of fire.

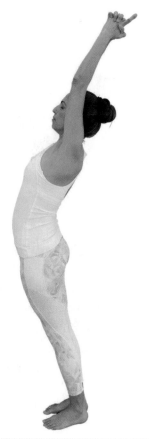

8. Forward Hang

Stand with your feet hip-distance apart. Inhale, and on the exhale, slowly bend forward, allowing your hands to drop toward your ankles. Bend your knees slightly and let your opposite hands rest in opposite elbows. Relax your head and soften your jaw.

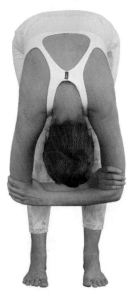

9. Standing Neck Turns with Yes and No

Stand in mountain pose and begin to chant the word *no* as you move the head side to side. Practice saying *no* out loud to the things that don't make your heart sing. Play around with different tones as you chant *no*. Practice for one minute. Then move the head up and down and chant *yes*. Practice saying *yes* to the things that light you up and open your heart chakra. Play around with different rhythms and tones as you chant *yes*. Continue for one minute.

10. Yoga Mudra

Feet are hip-distance apart. Interlace the fingers behind your back with the palms touching (if possible). Inhale and lift the head and chest up and stretch the arms away from your back. Exhale, bend the knees, and move the head toward the floor, raising the arms up toward the ceiling. Use a strap between the hands if the shoulders are tight.

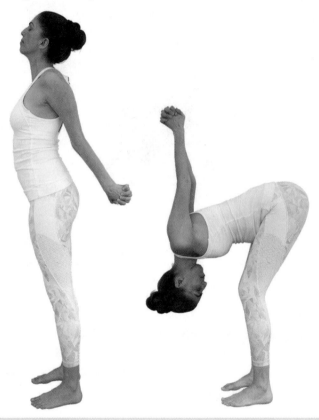

Sat Kriya for the Chakras

All the chakras work together even though many of the yoga sets in this book focus on one particular chakra. When you work on any one chakra, you are working on all of them. This kriya starts with the root chakra and moves the energy up to the crown chakra. It awakens, balances, and heals your chakra system and restores health, vitality, and mental focus. In each pose, you chant the mantra *Sat Nam*, which means, "I am truth and truth is my essence." The sound vibration from the mantra creates a high vibration in your chakra system and aligns your chakras with the infinite energy of the cosmos.

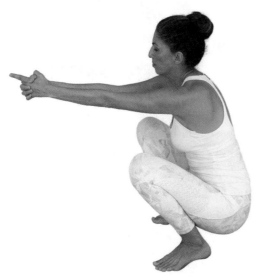

1. Root Chakra

Come into a squat with the soles of the feet touching the floor or resting on a blanket. Extend the arms in front of the heart chakra with the fingers interlaced and the index finger pointing forward. Pull in the navel and chant *Sat*. Relax the navel and chant *Nam*. Continue for one to three minutes.

Visualize a beautiful red light at the base of your spine with energy flowing down through the legs and feet into the earth. Visualize drawing energy and nourishment from the earth to your feet and legs.

2. Sacral Chakra

Lie on your stomach with the arms extended in front of you. Interlace the fingers and point the index fingers forward. Lift arms and legs off the floor and begin to chant *Sat Nam*. Continue for one to three minutes.

Visualize a beautiful orange light around your hips, low back, pelvis, and sex organs. Welcome more pleasure, excitement, and passion into your second chakra.

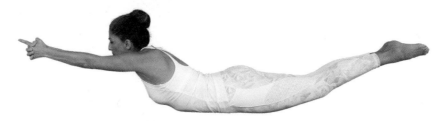

3. Navel Chakra

Sit in rock pose or easy pose and bring the hands to your navel point. Press the palms together with the fingers pointing away from you. Chant *Sat Nam* for one to three minutes.

Visualize a beautiful yellow light around your solar plexus and mid-back. Welcome the warm, radiant sun energy infusing you with power, energy, and vitality.

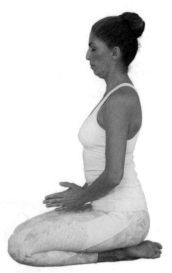

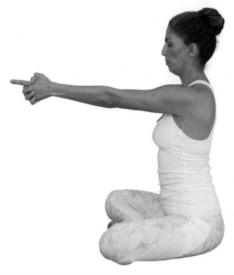

4. Heart Chakra

Sit in easy pose and bring the arms in front of the heart chakra. Interlace the fingers and point the index fingers forward. Chant *Sat Nam* for one to three minutes.

Visualize a beautiful green light around your heart chakra, flowing down your arms, hands, and shoulders. Welcome deeper feelings of love, acceptance, and compassion.

5. Throat Chakra

Sit on the heels and lower your body to the floor. Stretch the arms above your throat with the fingers interlaced and the index fingers pointing toward the sky. Variations include reclining on a bolster or blanket for support, keeping the legs straight out, or keeping the knees bent and the feet flat on the floor. Chant *Sat Nam* for one to three minutes.

Visualize a beautiful turquoise color around your throat, jaw, mouth, and ears. Welcome healing energy to your throat chakra so you fully express your truth and your creativity.

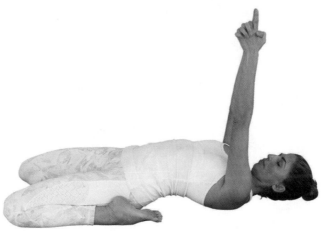

6. Third Eye Chakra

Come into child's pose and extend the arms in front with the palms touching and the thumbs interlaced. Chant *Sat Nam* for one to three minutes.

Visualize a beautiful indigo color around your eyes and forehead. Connect with your wisdom, light, and grace.

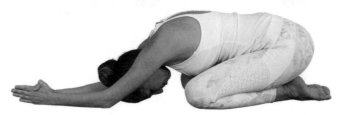

7. Crown Chakra

Come into shoulder stand or plow pose with the arms pointing toward the feet, fingers interlaced, and index fingers pointing. You can keep your hands on your lower back. Or, practice supported shoulder stand and place a block under the low back and lift the legs up.

Alternatively, practice bridge pose. And for plow pose, you can stack blankets under the feet and keep the hands on the low back. Chant *Sat Nam* for one to three minutes.

Visualize a beautiful purple light around the top of your head, connecting you with divine energy and consciousness. Welcome more bliss into your life.

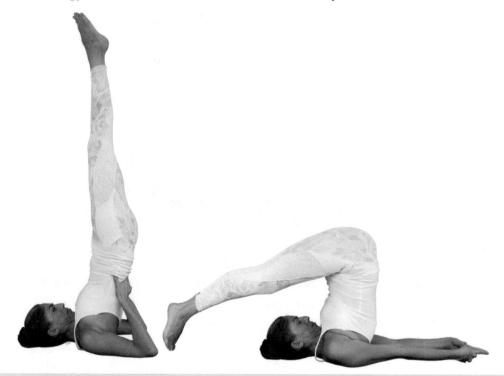

8. *The Aura*

Sit on the heels with the arms overhead and the palms together. Interlace the fingers except for the index fingers, which point straight up. To connect with your masculine energy, cross the right thumb over the left. To connect with your feminine energy, cross the left thumb over the right. Begin chanting *Sat Nam*. Powerfully chant *Sat* and pull the navel back toward the spine. Chant *Nam* as you relax and release the navel. Continue for one to three minutes.

Visualize a rainbow of colors along your spine, starting with red, orange, yellow, blue, violet, and purple. Visualize the lights as spiraling beams of energy moving through your system and filling your aura with strength, love, compassion, and joy.

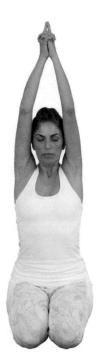

Relax *for fifteen minutes*

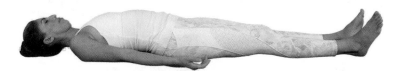

Rest on your back with the legs straight and the feet splayed out to the sides. Make sure you are warm and comfortable as you begin this relaxation. Soften the ankles, calves, and shins and let the thighs melt into the floor. Visualize a beautiful red color around your feet and legs infusing you with strength and stability. Draw in nurturing energy from Mother Earth. Relax your hips, thighs, and sex organs as you visualize a spiraling orange light balancing the energy at your sacral chakra. Welcome new levels of joy into your life as this orange light washes over you like waves in an ocean. Allow your breath to find its own natural rhythm while softening the navel area. Connect with your inner sun as you visualize a yellow light at your navel chakra restoring your confidence and energy. Relax the chest, shoulders, arms, and hands as you visualize a green light healing your heart chakra and filling you with unconditional love and acceptance. Soften the muscles in the neck and throat as you imagine a blue light around your throat chakra connecting you with your truth. Relax your entire face and soften the eyes as you see a spiraling violet light around your third eye chakra. Connect with your intuition and wisdom to guide you to serve the greater good. Relax your head as you visualize a thousand-petaled lotus of violet light around your crown chakra bringing you deep peace and relaxation.

Meditation to Balance the Chakras

This meditation is for handling the pressures of life, including information overload. As you practice this meditation, your breathing will change. Use your breath, the energy of prana, to carry you through. Keep your right arm stretched out parallel to the ground to align with the magnetic field of the earth. Your left hand is at your pituitary gland to balance the higher chakras. As discomfort arises, breathe deeply, notice it, and then let it go. Notice when you get caught up in the resistance (or in the story your mind is telling you), and then keep coming back to the breath.

Posture

Sit in easy pose with a straight spine. Put the fingers of the left hand on your forehead, touching your third eye point. Extend your right arm straight forward from your shoulder with the palm facing left. Close your eyes, hold the position, breathe slowly and deeply, meditate silently. Recharge your body with energy.

Eye Focus

Eyes are closed.

Breath

Slow, deep breaths.

Time

Practice for three to fifteen minutes.

To End

Inhale, hold your breath for five to ten seconds, and exhale. Repeat this sequence one more time. Then inhale, hold your breath for ten to fifteen seconds with your fingers interlocked over your head, and stretch your spine upward. Exhale and relax.

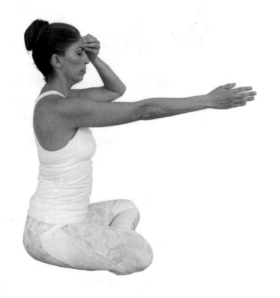

Meditation for Healing

This mantra has eight sounds that stimulate the flow of kundalini energy in the central channel. This healing meditation connects you to the divine energy of the universe so you feel connected and whole. As you chant, direct the healing energy to yourself and to those in your life who need support. Become aware of the healing energy around your hands and heart.

Posture

Sit in easy pose with a light neck lock.

Mudra

The elbows are bent by your sides and resting comfortably against the ribs. The forearms are perpendicular to the floor, with the hands extended out at a 45-degree angle from the center of the body. The palms are perfectly flat, facing up; hands are bent back at the wrists. Fingers are kept side by side, except the thumbs are spread wide from the four fingers.

Eye Focus

Eyes are closed. Mentally visualize the person or persons you are wanting to heal as you send this energy to them for their well-being.

Mantra

Ra Ma Da Sa, Sa Say So Hung (Sun, Moon, Earth, Infinite Spirit)

   This mantra taps into the energies of the sun, moon, earth, and Infinite Spirit to bring deep healing. Pull the navel point on the first *Sa* and on *Hung*. Chant one complete cycle of the entire mantra with each breath. Then deeply inhale and repeat.

Breath

Inhale after each repetition.

Time

Practice for ten to thirty minutes.

Meditation for Healing (continued)

To End

Inhale deeply and hold the breath as you offer a healing prayer to all those in your life who need support. Visualize them engulfed in a healing white light and completely healed. Then exhale and relax.

Music Recommendations

Ajeet Kaur, *Haseya*

Gurudass Kaur, *Lovingly*

Snatuam Kaur, *Grace*

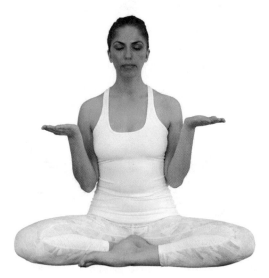

Going Forward

I hope you have enjoyed the process of learning about yourself and your chakras and that this has been a voyage of self-discovery. The intention of this book is to connect you more deeply with your true nature and to rejoice in who you are in this moment. All the practices in this book are meant to be seen as self-care for your system rather than self-improvement. All you need is already within you, and these practices help connect you with your inner strengths.

You may be wondering how to get started or how to stay committed now that you've worked your way through the book. I recommend going back and diving into the chapter that most resonates with you and sparks your interest and curiosity. Excitement is important when you are starting something new. Practice some of the exercises from that chapter on a daily basis. Some days, practice for five minutes, and other days, practice for thirty to forty-five minutes. Often, I devote a month to a chakra and commit to a daily practice of nurturing it. I start small with a five-minute meditation, and when that becomes easy, I lengthen the time and build confidence, one small step at a time.

Be compassionate with yourself as you start these practices, and continue to enrich and deepen your understanding of how your chakra system works. Know that there will be many starts and stops—that is part of the journey, so let go of perfection. Identify obstacles that may arise and write down strategies to counter them. You can be sure that challenges will show up, but you can be prepared in order to overcome them.

If possible, recruit a few kindred spirits to join you on this journey; we commit more deeply when we cocreate and share experiences with others. Create a chakra tribe of peers who will support and encourage you as you grow. May you be blessed with health and happiness as you continue to unlock the power of your chakras.

May you be safe.
May you be healthy.
May you be happy.
May you live with ease.

Bibliography

Achor, Shawn. *The Happiness Advantage: The Seven Principals of Positive Psychology That Fuel Success and Performance at Work*. New York: Crown Business, 2010.

Allen, David. *Getting Things Done: The Art of Stress-Free Productivity*. New York: Penguin Books, 2001.

Adams, Kathleen. "A Short Course in Journal Writing: It's Easy to W.R.I.T.E." *Center for Journal Therapy*. Accessed January 18, 2022. https://journaltherapy.com/lets-journal/a-short-course-in-journal-writing/.

Avalon, Arthur. *The Serpent Power: The Secrets of Tantric & Shaktic Yoga*. New York: Dover Publications, 1974.

Bhajan, Yogi. *The Aquarian Teacher Level One Instructor Manual*. Espanola, NM: Kundaini Research Institute, 2010.

———. *The Aquarian Teacher Level One Instructor Textbook*. Espanola, NM: Kundaini Research Institute, 2010.

Bradshaw, John. *Home Coming: Reclaiming and Healing Your Inner Child*. New York: Bantam Books, 1990.

Brennan, Ann Barbara. *Hands of Light: A Guide to Healing Through the Human Energy Field*. New York: Bantam Books, 1987.

Chopra, Deepak. *What Are You Hungry For? The Chopra Solution to Permanent Weight Loss, Well-Being, and Lightness of Soul*. New York: Harmony Books, 2013.

Clear, James. *Atomic Habits: An Easy & Proven Way to Build Good Habits & Break Bad Ones*. New York: Avery, 2018.

Covey, R. Stephen. *The 7 Habits of Highly Effective People: Powerful Lessons in Personal Change*. New York: Simon & Shuster, 1989.

Dale, Cyndi. *Complete Book of Chakras: Your Definitive Source of Energy Center Knowledge for Health, Happiness, and Spiritual Evolution*. Woodbury, MN: Llewellyn Publications, 2016.

———. *Energetic Boundaries: How to Stay Protected and Connected in Work, Love, and Life*. Boulder, CO: Sounds True, 2011.

———. *Llewellyn's Little Book of Chakras*. Woodbury, MN: Llewellyn Publications, 2007.

Desikachar, T. K. V. *The Heart of Yoga: Developing A Personal Practice*. Rochester, VT: Inner Traditions International, 1995.

Ekman, Paul. "Universal Emotions." *Paul Ekman Group*. Accessed January 18, 2022. https://www.paulekman.com/universal-emotions/.

Garvin, David A., and Michael A. Roberto. "What You Don't Know About Making Decisions." *Harvard Business Review* 79, no. 8 (September 2001): 108–116.

Hanson, Rick. *Hardwiring Happiness: The New Brain Science of Contentment, Calm, and Confidence*. New York: Harmony Books, 2013.

Hanson, Rick, and Forrest Hanson. *Resilient: How to Grow an Unshakable Core of Calm, Strength, and Happiness*. New York: Harmony, 2018.

Hendriksen, Ellen. *How to Be Yourself: Quiet Your Inner Critic and Rise Above Social Anxiety*. New York: St. Martin Griffin, 2018.

Johari, Harish. *Chakras: Energy Centers of Transformation*. Rochester, VT: Destiny Books, 2000.

Judith, Anodea. *Chakra Balancing Kit: A Guide to Healing and Awakening Your Energy Body*. Boulder, CO: Sounds True, 2003.

———. *Chakras Made Easy: Seven Keys to Awakening and Healing the Energy Body*. Carlsbad, CA: Hay House, 2016.

Judith, Anodea. *Chakra Yoga*. Woodbury, MN: Llewellyn Publications, 2015.

———. *Wheels of Life: A User's Guide to the Chakra System*. St. Paul, MN: Llewellyn Publications, 1987.

Judith, Anodea, and Selene Vega. *The Sevenfold Journey: Reclaiming Mind, Body, & Spirit Through the Chakras*. Berkeley, CA: Crossing Press, 1993.

Judith, Anodea, and Lion Goodman. *Creating on Purpose: The Spiritual Technology of Manifesting Through the Chakras*. Boulder, CO: Sounds True, 2012.

Khalsa, Kaur Gurmukh. *The Eight Human Talents: Restore Balance and Serenity Within You with Kundalini Yoga*. New York: Harper, 1997.

Khalsa, Kaur Hari. *A Women's Book of Meditation: Discovering the Power of a Peaceful Mind*. New York: Avery, 2006.

Khalsa, Kaur Harijot. *Reaching Me in Me: Kundalini Yoga As Taught By Yogi Bhajan*. New Mexico: Kundalini Research Institute, 2001.

———. *Self-Knowledge: Kundalini Yoga As Taught By Yogi Bhajan*. New Mexico: Kundalini Research Institute, 2001.

Khalsa, Kaur Sat Purkh. *Transformation: Seeds of Change for the Aquarian Age*. New Mexico: Kundalini Research Institute, 2010.

Khalsa, Kaur Shakta. *Kundalini Yoga: Unlock Your Inner Potential Through Life-Changing Exercise.* London and New York: Dorling Kindersley, 2001.

Khalsa, Singh Guru Dharam, and Darryl O'Keeffe. *The Kundalini Yoga Experience: Bringing Body, Mind and Spirit Together.* New York: Fireside, 2002.

Khalsa, Singh Dharma, and Cameron Stauth. *Meditation as Medicine: Activate the Power of Your Natural Healing Force.* New York: Atria Paperback, 2001.

Khalsa, Singh Gurucharan. *Kundalini Yoga: Sadhana Guidelines.* New Mexico: Kundalini Research Institute, 2007.

Khalsa, Guru Meher. *Senses of the Soul: Emotional Therapy for Strength, Healing and Guidance.* New Mexico: Kundalini Research Institute, 2013.

Khalsa, Singh Nirvair. *The Ten Light Bodies of Consciousness: A Guide to Self-Discovery and Self-Enlightenment.* Anchorage, AK: NSK Production, 1994.

Kubler-Ross, Elisabeth, and Kessler David. *On Grief & Grieving: Finding the Meaning of Grief Through the Five Stages of Loss.* New York: Scribner, 2005.

Le Page, Joseph, and Lilian Le Page. *Yoga Toolbox for Teachers and Students: Yoga Posture Cards for Harmonizing All Dimensions of Your Being.* Integrative Yoga Therapy, 2015.

Muktibodhananda, Swami. *Hatha Yoga Pradipika.* Munger, Bihar, India: Yoga Publications Trust, 1985.

Neff, Kristin. *Self-Compassion: The Proven Power of Being Kind to Yourself.* New York: William Morrow, 2011.

Neff, Kristin, and Christopher Germer. *The Mindful Self-Compassion Workbook: A Proven Way to Accept Yourself, Build Inner Strength, and Thrive.* New York and London: The Guilford Press, 2018.

Rosenberg, Marshall. *Nonviolent Communication: A Language of Life.* Encinitas, CA: Puddle Dancer Press, 2015.

Saraswati, Swami Satyananda. *Kundalini Tantra.* Munger, Bihar, India: Yoga Publications Trust, 1984.

Walker, Matthew. *Why We Sleep: Unlocking the Power of Sleep and Dreams.* New York: Scribner, 2017.

Wauters, Ambika. *The Complete Guide to Chakras: Unleash the Positive Power Within.* New York: Barron's, 2002.

Wilson, Larry, and Hersch Wilson. *Play to Win: Choosing Growth Over Fear in Work and Life.* Austin, TX: Bard Press, 1998.

Index

To Write to the Author

If you wish to contact the author or would like more information about this book, please write to the author in care of Llewellyn Worldwide Ltd. and we will forward your request. Both the author and the publisher appreciate hearing from you and learning of your enjoyment of this book and how it has helped you. Llewellyn Worldwide Ltd. cannot guarantee that every letter written to the author can be answered, but all will be forwarded. Please write to:

Masuda Mohamadi
℅ Llewellyn Worldwide
2143 Wooddale Drive
Woodbury, MN 55125-2989
Please enclose a self-addressed stamped envelope for reply,
or $1.00 to cover costs. If outside the U.S.A., enclose
an international postal reply coupon.

Many of Llewellyn's authors have websites with additional information and resources. For more information, please visit our website at http://www.llewellyn.com.